Bi & Gi Publishers

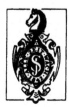

Current Topics in Rehabilitation
Series Editor : R. Corsico M.D.

Titles in the series:

Cardiopulmonary Rehabilitation

Edited by: C. Rampulla, C. Fracchia, N. Ambrosino

Foreword by R. Corsico
With 24 figures and 22 tables

Springer-Verlag London Ltd.

C. Rampulla   Clinica del Lavoro Foundation, Institute of Care and Research, Medical Center of
               Rehabilitation, Montescano (Pavia) Italy
C. Fracchia   Clinica del Lavoro Foundation, Institute of Care and Research, Medical Center of
               Rehabilitation, Montescano (Pavia) Italy
N. Ambrosino   Clinica del Lavoro Foundation, Institute of Care and Research, Medical Center of
               Rehabilitation, Montescano (Pavia) Italy

Series Editor:
R. Corsico   Clinica del Lavoro Foundation, Institute of Care and Research, Medical Center of
               Rehabilitation, Montescano (Pavia), Italy

ISBN 978-1-4471-3781-8

British Library Cataloguing in Publication Data
Cardiopulmonary rehabilitation (Current Topics in Rehabilitation Series)
ISBN 978-1-4471-3781-8

Library of Congress Cataloging in Publication Data
Cardiopulmonary rehabilitation / edited by C. Rampulla, C. Fracchia, N. Ambrosino: foreword by R.
Corsico: with figures and tables.
p. cm. -- (Current topics in rehabilitation). Includes bibliographical references and index.
ISBN 978-1-4471-3781-8   ISBN 978-1-4471-3779-5 (eBook)
DOI 10.1007/978-1-4471-3779-5

1. Lungs -- Diseases, Obstructive -- Patients -- Rehabilitation.
2. Cardiopulmonary system -- Diseases -- Patients -- Rehabilitation.
I. Rampulla C. (Ciro), 1942 - II. Fracchia C. (Claudio), 1951 - III. Ambrosino N. (Nicola) 1948.
IV. Series RC776.O3C37 1993   616.2'0046 -- dc 20   93-13742 CIP

© 1993 Springer-Verlag London
Originally published by Bi & Gi Publishers in 1993
Softcover reprint of the hardcover 1st edition 1993

Foreword

Pulmonary rehabilitation has for a long time been considered as a younger sister of pneumology. On the contrary, it has the dignity of being an autonomous discipline, for two reasons: it uses specific methods of evaluation and treatment, not derived from pneumology, and it has a "contra science".

A "contra science" is a mirror discipline which provides information to our discipline from which it takes information useful for its development. The contra science of pulmonary rehabilitation is not pneumology but respiratory physiology. The rehabilitation of the nineties is completely different from the earlier years, starting with the definition.

Respiratory rehabilitation is defined as "long term evaluation and therapy". This definition is remarkably different from the old ones and implies that evaluation techniques and treatment strategies are the main body of this discipline. Consequently respiratory rehabilitation is not merely exercise. In the last years many problems associated with symptoms such as dyspnoea and exercise limitation, with muscle fatigue and ventilatory failure, have been elucidated. Consequently new therapeutic strategies have been elaborated in which rehabilitation has a main role. Classic manoeuvres such as bronchial drainage, breathing exercise and physical exercise training remain as weapons in the treatment of respiratory diseases, but new techniques, such as respiratory muscle training and non-invasive mechanical ventilation and have been developed. Finally, patients who have undergone mechanical ventilation by tracheostomy and need long, term weaning are now patients who can be submitted for rehabilitation.

All these considerations were enough to stimulate an attempt to categorize such changes and to promote an international workshop in 1990 to update our knowledge of cardiopulmonary rehabilitation. This book, which reports the proceedings of that meeting, is the result of such an effort.

RENATO CORSICO

Preface

Only long term oxygen therapy prolongs survival in hypoxemic COPD patients. Consequently improving dyspnoea and exercise tolerance is a main goal of the treatment of these patients. During the last few years there have been considerable changes in the field of pulmonary rehabilitation. Respiratory rehabilitation programs are widely accepted as important in the management of patients with chronic obstructive pulmonary diseases. Several studies have alluded to the benefits of rehabilitation, but only a few have been prospective randomized or controlled, and cost/ benefit ratios, both for the individual and for the community, in comparison with costs and benefits of conventional care, are still to be defined. Although pulmonary rehabilitation is still regarded more as an art than a science, many new concepts, both from the theoretical and from the practical point of view, have been underlined. Patient selection can be considered as one of these new concepts. In fact, in comparison to the previous indications which included age, functional status, definite pathological status and so on, today the only contra indication that should be considered is poor compliance to treatment. Functional status was a rigid frame work in which to include patients to be submitted to pulmonary rehabilitation: hypercapnic respiratory failure is now considered as a field of intervention in the light of the new knowledge of the pump system, respiratory muscles and respiratory muscle fatigue.

Therapy for the relief of dyspnoea is primarily aimed at reducing reversible airflow obstruction with bronchodilator drugs, preventing or promptly treating infections also with bronchial drainage techniques. Exercise training has the potential to improve exercise endurance and reduce exertional dyspnoea. Different psychophysical techniques may be used to measure the sensation of dyspnoea. Interval scales like the visual analogue scale and Borg's scale are easy to use and show relatively good reproducibility in healthy subjects and in patients with chronic respiratory diseases.

Limited exercise capacity is the prime feature of chronic airflow obstruction and results mostly from pulmonary limitation, especially related to the abnormal mechanical characteristics of the respiratory system. Exercise testing evaluation is difficult because various investigators use a variety of protocols probably due to a lack in recommended guidelines for the exercise testing of normal and in patients.

Specific training exercises for strength and endurance improve performance in ventilatory muscles.

For the rehabilitation of the respiratory patient, metabolic balance and maintenance of nutrition appear no less important than ventilation itself because the two are inextricably related.

Ventilatory failure can result from the impairment of each component of the ventilatory pump or from the interaction between an injured component and the rest of the ventilatory machinery.

Inspiratory muscle fatigue may be a cause of hypercapnic respiratory failure in COPD, in restrictive lung and chest wall diseases and in neuromuscular diseases. Regardless of the mechanism, rest should be the best treatment for fatigued inspiratory muscles. Inspiratory muscles can be unloaded by the application of cyclic negative pressure to the chest wall by lung or cuirass and poncho wrap ventilators. Non-invasive intermittent positive pressure ventilation applied through a nasal mask has been shown to be useful in the treatment of chronic respiratory failure.

When acute respiratory failure ensures the admission to an intensive care unit it can be life-saving but it can also create a ventilator-dependent patient. Since hospital charges for ventilator-assisted patients are very expensive and intensive care unit beds are relatively insufficient, ventilator-dependent patients need a less expensive structure that can take care of their management and their discharge from the hospital to home, or alternatively, to community sites.

The goals of a so-called "subintensive respiratory care unit" do not finish in the hospital but extend to home care.

The concept of home care for respiratory diseases, however, is still related exclusively to the improved chances of survival and application of specialized technology such as mechanical ventilation or oxygen therapy.

This book provides an up to date review of these subjects and indicates the many areas in need of further investigation. We are grateful to the contributors for presenting these most provocative works and thoughts.

C. FRACCHIA, C. RAMPULLA, N. AMBROSINO

Contents

Respiratory Failure

Contributors

AMBROSINO N.

Division of Pulmonary Disease, Clinica del Lavoro Foundation, Institute of Care and Research, Medical Center of Rehabilitation, Montescano, Pavia, Italy

APPENDINI L.

Division of Pulmonary Disease, Clinica del Lavoro Foundation, Institute of Care and Research, Medical Center of Rehabilitation, Veruno, Italy

BRAGHIROLI A.

Division of Pulmonary Disease, Clinica del Lavoro Foundation, Institute of Care and Research, Medical Center of Rehabilitation, Veruno, Italy

CABROL C.

Department of Cardiovascular Surgery, Paris VI, France

CERRETELLI P.

Physiology Laboratories, University of Geneva, Switzerland

CORSICO R.

Division of Pulmonary Disease, Clinica del Lavoro Foundation, Institute of Care and Research, Medical Center of Rehabilitation, Montescano, Pavia, Italy

COX N.

Department Pulmonary Diseases, Dekkerswald Medical Center, University of Nijmegen, The Netherlands

DARDES N.

Fatebenefratelli General Hospital, Isola Tiberina, Rome, Italy

DEKHUIJZEN R.

Department Pulmonary Diseases, Dekkerswald Medical Center, University of Nijmegen, The Netherlands

DONNER C.F.

Division of Pulmonary Disease, Clinica del Lavoro Foundation, Institute of Care and Research, Medical Center of Rehabilitation, Veruno, Italy

FERRANTI R.D.

Gayl ord Rehabilitation Hospital, Center for Breathing Disorders, Wallingford, CT, USA

Yale University Medical School, Section of Pulmonary Disease, New Haven, USA

FITTING J.W.

Division of Pneumology, Department of Internal Medicine, Chuv, Lausanne, Switzerland

XII

FOLGERING H.
Department Pulmonary Diseases, Dekkerswald Medical Center, University of Nijmegen, The Netherlands

FORNI G.
Division of Cardiology, Clinica del Lavoro Foundation, Institute of Care and Research, Medical Center of Rehabilitation, Montescano, Pavia, Italy

FRACCHIA C.
Division of Pulmonary Disease, Clinica del Lavoro Foundation, Institute of Care and Research, Medical Center of Rehabilitation, Montescano, Pavia, Italy

FRANCHINI M.
Division of Cardiology, Clinica del Lavoro Foundation, Institute of Care and Research, Medical Center of Rehabilitation, Montescano, Pavia, Italy

GOLDSTEIN R.S.
West Park Hospital, Mount Sinai Hospital, Department of Medicine, University of Toronto, Ontario, Canada

GORT E.H.
West Park Hospital, Mount Sinai Hospital, Department of Medicine, University of Toronto, Ontario, Canada

GRASSI B.
ITBA-CNR, Milano

HERWAARDEN C.V.
Department Pulmonary Diseases, Dekkerswald Medical Center, University of Nijmegen, The Netherlands

HOWARD P.
Department of Medicine and Pharmacology, University of Sheffield, Royal Hallamshire Hospital, Sheffield, United Kingdom

LACHMAN A.
Clinique de pneumologie, Hôpital Universitaire Saint-Pierre, Bruxelles, Belgium

LUSUARDI M.
Division of Pulmonary Disease, Clinica del Lavoro Foundation, Institute of Care and Research, Medical Center of Rehabilitation, Veruno, Italy

MALFA R.
Gaylord Rehabilitation Hospital, Center for Breathing Disorders, Wallingford, CT, USA

MARCONI C.
ITBA-CNR, Milano

MEYER M.
Max Planck Institute Exp. Med., Göttingen, Germany

MILIC-EMILI J.
Meakins-Christie Laboratories, McGill University, Montreal, Quebec, Canada

MORPURGO M.
Department of Cardiology, San Carlo Borromeo Hospital, Milan, Italy

MUIR J.F.
Service de Pneumologie, Hôpital de Bois-Guillaume, CHU Rouen, France

PELLICCIOTTI L.
Fatebenefratelli General Hospital, Isola Tiberina, Rome, Italy

RAMPULLA C.
Division of Pulmonary Disease, Clinica del Lavoro Foundation, Institute of Care and Research, Medical Center of Rehabilitation, Montescano, Pavia, Italy

RE M.A.
Fatebenefratelli General Hospital, Isola Tiberina, Rome, Italy

RIEU M.
Physiology Laboratories of Paris V, France

ROCHESTER D.F.
E. Cato Drash Professor of Medicine, Division of Pulmonary and Critical Care Medicine, Department of Internal Medicine, University of Virginia School of Medicine, Charlottesville, Virginia, USA

ROSSI A.
Respiratory Division, O.C.M., U.S.L. 25, Verona, and Department of Internal Medicine, University of Verona, Italy

RUSSO L.
Fatebenefratelli General Hospital, Isola Tiberina, Rome, Italy

SANNA A.
Clinique de pneumologie, Hôpital Universitaire Saint-Pierre, Bruxelles, Belgium

SERGYSELS R.
Clinique de pneumologie, Hôpital Universitaire Saint-Pierre, Bruxelles, Belgium

STEWART A.G.
Department of Medicine and Pharmacology, University of Sheffield, Royal Hallamshire Hospital, Sheffield, United Kingdom

TORBICKI A.
Department of Hypertension and Angiology, Academy of Medicine, Warszawa, Poland

TRAMARIN R.

Division of Cardiology, Clinica del Lavoro Foundation, Institute of Care and Research, Medical Center of Rehabilitation, Montescano, Pavia, Italy

VULTERINI S.

Fatebenefratelli General Hospital, Isola Tiberina, Rome, Italy

ZACCARIA E.

Division of Pulmonary Disease, Clinica del Lavoro Foundation, Institute of Care and Research, Medical Center of Rehabilitation, Veruno, Italy

ZACCARIA S.

Division of Pulmonary Disease, Clinica del Lavoro Foundation, Institute of Care and Research, Medical Center of Rehabilitation, Veruno, Italy

ZANABONI S.

Division of Pulmonary Disease, Clinica del Lavoro Foundation, Institute of Care and Research, Medical Center of Rehabilitation, Veruno, Italy

Rehabilitation Programs

1. Old and New in Pulmonary Rehabilitation

D.F. ROCHESTER

E. Cato Drash Professor of Medicine, Division of Pulmonary and Critical Care Medicine, Department of Internal Medicine, University of Virginia School of Medicine, Charlottesville, Virginia, USA

Introduction

Pulmonary rehabilitation for patients with chronic lung disease traditionally included interventions designed to improve the position of the diaphragm, breathing exercises based on pursed lips breathing, relaxation, and enhancement of abdominal excursion, and physical exercise training. Newer training programs have been designed specifically to enhance the endurance of the respiratory muscles. This review summarizes the results of these interventions, especially with regard to their effects on respiratory muscle function, capacity for physical exercise, and ability to conduct activities of daily living.

Diaphragmatic Position and Excursion

Head down position

Barach and Beck studied 24 patients with "pulmonary emphysema", some of whom were hypercapnic.[1] Adopting a 16 degrees head down position reduced minute ventilation by 23%, with no significant effect on $PaCO_2$ or SaO_2. Diaphragmatic excursion during quiet breathing increased from less than 1.5 cm upright to 3.5 cm head down. The authors reported that dyspnea was markedly reduced.

Gayrard et al.[2] studied 13 patients with COPD (RV 200% predicted, TLC 120% predicted). The head down position displaced the resting diaphragm about 3 cm more cephalad, with no change in either the tidal or the maximal excursion.

Abdominal weights used in supine or head down positions had similar but generally lesser effects.

Artificial pneumoperitoneum

Artificial pneumoperitoneum improved vital capacity (VC), maximum breathing capacity (MBC), $PaCO_2$ and diaphragmatic excursion in 23 patients with severe COPD.[3-5] The MBC averaged 29±9 l/min prior to pneumoperitoneum, and 36±12 l/min afterward (P<0.001). Maximal diaphragmatic excursion was only 1 to 2 cm prior to pneumoperitoneum, and increased by about 3 cm after the procedure. The volume of air injected into the peritoneum was generally much less than required to collapse pulmonary cavities caused by tuberculosis.[3] About half of the patients were "clinically improved" or had less dyspnea when walking,[3,5] and one recovered dramatically from severe acute hypercapnic respiratory failure.

Breathing Exercises

The term "breathing exercises" refers to a variety of techniques, including pursed-lip breathing,[7,8] diaphragmatic breathing,[9] as well as variants which also include relaxation and increased abdominal excursion.[10-12] The primary goal of breathing exercises is to develop a slower, deeper pattern of breathing, especially in patients with chronic obstructive pulmonary disease (COPD).

Immediate effects

When patients with COPD adopted a slow, deep pattern of breathing while at rest, the respiratory rate typically fell by about 45%, the tidal volume increased by about 65%, and minute ventilation fell by 15%. As a result, alveolar ventilation increased from 45% to 57% of total minute ventilation, $PaCO_2$ fell by 2 to 5 torr, and PaO_2 increased by 1 to 5 torr.[7,8,13-15]

During exercise the relative changes in rate, tidal volume and minute ventilation were similar,[7,14] but there was no significant change in blood gas composition.

Bellemare and Grassino showed that slow, deep breathing could cause the diaphragmatic tension-time index to move into a range which would cause fatigue, if the effort were to be sustained.[16]

Breathing exercise training

Three reports[9-11] describe the results of breathing exercise training for 3 to 12 weeks in a total of 61 COPD patients. Respiratory rate fell by 30%, tidal volume increased by 35%, and maximal ventilation (voluntary or exercise) increased by

22%. After training, $PaCO_2$ was 3 to 7 torr lower, and there were concomitant improvements in PaO_2 or SaO_2. Modest improvements in VC, FEV_1 and RV/TLC were also noted. The effect of breathing exercise training on maximal exercise performance is negligible.[11,17] However, when 3 weeks of breathing exercise training was superimposed on the last 3 weeks of a 9 week physical exercise training program, the maximal oxygen consumption was 30% higher than one with the same period of physical training without the breathing exercise.[12]

Breathing exercise training improved the maximal excursion of the diaphragm and respiratory muscle strength. In 3 studies,[9-11] the average baseline excursion was 2.6 cm, and it increased to 5.5 cm after training (P < 0.001).

The PEmax increased by 16%, and Pdi max by 30%.[18] Abdominal sit-up exercises increased Pdi max by 15% (P=NS), but exercising by using the diaphragm to lift weights on the abdomen did not change Pdi, maximal inspiratory flow rate or inspiratory capacity in normal subjects.[19]

Physical Exercise Training

Physical exercise training improves ventilatory or inspiratory muscle endurance in patients with cystic fibrosis, by about 50%.[20,21] In COPD the results are less impressive. A review of older literature led to the conclusion that approximately 40% of COPD patients improved their MVV by 10% or more with physical exercise training.[22] However, other studies have shown that physical exercise training leads to little or no change in the inspiratory muscle function of patients with COPD.[23-25]

The effect of upper extremity exercise on the respiratory muscles illustrates another issue which bears on respiratory muscle endurance. Unsupported arm exercise forces the respiratory muscles to assist in stabilizing the torso and thus decreases their contribution to ventilation.[26] Even normal subjects may experience irregular breathing patterns, dyspnea and shortened exercise tolerance during upper extremity exercise.

Respiratory Muscle Training

Objectives

The obvious goals for respiratory muscle training are to increase the strength and endurance of these muscles, as well as ventilatory endurance. Probably more important for the quality of life, inspiratory muscle training should improve the capacity for activities of daily living (ADL), with less dyspnea. Finally, a goal for hypercapnic patients might be to increase the tidal volume, so as to stabilize or improve the $PaCO_2$.

Training techniques

Strength

The strength of the inspiratory and expiratory muscles can be substantially increased by performing repetitive maximal static inspiratory and expiratory efforts.[27] The value of strength training by itself has not been explored, but one can hypothesize that it might benefit in two ways. First, muscle strength has some bearing on muscle endurance.[16,28] Second, strengthening the respiratory muscles might improve the capacity for activities like unsupported arm exercise, where the non-ventilatory component of respiratory muscle function competes with their ventilatory function.[26]

Endurance: hyperpnea

Regimens designed to improve ventilatory endurance are based on hyperpnea. Both ways of achieving isocapnic hyperpnea have significant practical limitations. Leith and Bradley[27] initiated the technique of voluntary isocapnic hyperpnea (VIH), and others have used it with modifications.[21,29-32] The problem with this approach is that it is cumbersome to hyperventilate and maintain $PaCO_2$ at baseline values. The alternative is physical exercise training, which is a more physiologic way to attain isocapnic hyperpnea. One limitation of this approach is that patients may not be able to exercise adequately for a variety of reasons, including cardiovascular, circulatory and neuromuscular disease.

In exercise training, it is important that the level of minute ventilation that is achieved during exercise is high enough to provide an adequate training stress. In VIH regimens, subjects are required to breathe at 50 to 70% of VEmax or MVV. It would be of interest to determine how long patients can sustain exercise that requires that level of ventilation, and the extent to which they use their respiratory muscles for non-ventilatory functions during exercise.

Endurance: inspiratory loading

Training the inspiratory muscles by requiring the subject to inspire against a load is appealing because it is relatively simple to do. Both inspiratory flow-resistive (IFRL) and inspiratory threshold loads (ITL) have been used. Usually the IFRL are not linear, because the device uses a fixed or variable orifice.[33-36] In that event, the inspiratory pressure increases exponentially instead of linearly, as the inspiratory flow rate increases.

With ITL the subject is required to overcome a weight or the force of a spring in order to initiate inspiratory flow.[37-39] Once flow has been initiated, the load remains constant, no matter how high or low the inspiratory flow rate is. The magnitude of the load can be adjusted by adding or subtracting weights, or by adjusting the compression of the spring.

For proper use of either IFRL or ITL, it is imperative to control the pattern of breathing. The objective of training with an inspiratory load is to increase the inspiratory pressure needed to inspire a breath (Pbreath), and to hold that pressure for about 40% of the breath. Belman has shown that subjects inspiring through an IFRL will develop a lower Pbreath with a small orifice than with a large one, provided they inspire slowly through the smaller orifice.[40] This effect is magnified by the alinear resistance, because a higher inspiratory flow rate more than offsets the advantage of a larger orifice. The ITL has the advantage of fixing the load independent of inspiratory flow rate. However, if one inspires a given tidal volume rapidly, then the preset load is endured for only a brief part of the total breath cycle.

Duration of training

The duration of respiratory muscle training was 4 to 6 weeks in most studies. During this time, the subject trained for 15 to 20 minutes per session, with 2 or 3 sessions per day, for 5 to 7 days per week. Most of the training benefit accrued in the first 4 to 8 weeks,[37,41] but training for a longer period offered modest additional benefits.[42,43]

Evaluation of endurance

Testing for endurance generally involves determining how many brief submaximal efforts, separated by brief rest periods, can be repeated. To this end, some investigators[27,29-32] use the maximal sustainable ventilatory capacity (MSVC). An increase in MSVC is considered to represent an increase in respiratory muscle endurance, provided there is no change in airway resistance. Others have defined inspiratory muscle endurance in terms of the highest resistive or threshold load that can be sustained for 10 min, or by the ventilatory endurance time in the presence of a submaximal inspiratory flow-resistive or threshold load.[33-43]

The dependence of inspiratory muscle endurance on muscle strength is apparent from examination of the pressure-time index. This index is the product of Pbreath/PImax and Ti/Ttot.[16,28] Thus, increasing PImax might increase ventilatory endurance as well as endurance for inspiratory loads. It has been shown that the maximal voluntary ventilation (MVV) is dependent on respiratory muscle strength,[44] but inspiratory loading training which increases PImax and endurance for the load does not seem to increase MSVC (Table I). This conclusion might be overturned if more data were available.

Results of training

Endurance

The effects of physical exercise (EXC), voluntary isocapnic hyperpnea (VIH) and inspiratory loading training (ILT) on the MSVC are summarized in Table I.

The two regimens based on hyperpnea, EXC and VIH, led to significant improvement in the MSVC, but IRL training did not. However, it should be noted that the number of IRL trained patients whose MSVC was tested was small, and their baseline MSVC was much lower than in the other groups. Moreover, despite lack of effect on MSVC, these patients did exhibit increased endurance for the inspiratory load.

Other evidence supports the concept that IRL training really does improve inspiratory muscle endurance. For example, IFRL training enabled patients to tolerate loads several times higher than prior to training,[17,24,34,43,45-48] and also decreased inspiratory muscle susceptibility to fatigue, based on electromyographic criteria.[41,42,45] In addition, IFRL and ITL double the ventilatory endurance time for breathing against the load.[33,37,39,41,43]

Weaning from mechanical ventilation

Two COPD patients underwent VIH training while recovering from acute respiratory failure, and increases in their MSVC were associated with successful discontinuation of ventilator support.[49] IFRL training helped 12 of 27 patients to wean from mechanical ventilation.[50] In the weaned group, PImax increased by 38%, whereas patients whose PImax increased by less than 10% failed to wean.

Strength

There are no data about the effects of VIH training on respiratory muscle strength in patients. Inspiratory loading training increases PImax (Table II), provided the training stimulus is large enough. A number of reports[33-39] were analyzed to quantify the inspiratory load in terms of its effect on Pbreath/PImax during the training periods. When training Pbreath/PImax averaged 45%, PImax increased by 35%.

Table I. Effect of inspiratory muscle training regimens on maximal sustainable ventilatory capacity (MSVC) in patients with COPD or cystic fibrosis.

Regimen (N)*	Before	MSVC(l/min)** After	%change
EXC (43)	62	71	15
VIH (40)	47	63	35
ILT (26)	30	30	1
CTRL (54)	44	46	5

* EXC = physical exercise, VIH = voluntary isocapnic hyperpnea, ILT = inspiratory loading training, CTRL = control, non-trained patients.
** Data compiled from references 20,21,23,29-32,35,38,45. The mean values from these studies were averaged, weighted according to the number of subjects in each group.

Table II. Effect of inspiratory loading training on inspiratory muscle strength (PImax) in patients with acute respiratory failure or COPD.

| Group (N)* | PImax (cmH$_2$O)** | | |
	Before	After	% change
ARF (27)	-37	-46	24
COPD (64)	-62	-74	20
CTRL (60)	-54	-58	7

* ARF = acute respiratory failure; COPD = chronic obstructive pulmonary disease; CTRL = control, non-trained COPD patients.
** Data compiled from references 33-39,50. The mean values from these studies were averaged, weighted according to the number of subjects in each group.

When Pbreath/PImax averaged 12%, PImax increased by only 7%. It appears that training Pbreath should exceed 30% PImax to achieve the desired result.

Exercise, ADL and dyspnea

The most consistent effect of inspiratory muscle training, using either VIH or ITL, is an increase in steady-state bicycle exercise endurance time. Exercise endurance time increased by 64% in 69 trained COPD patients, as compared to a 31% increase in control, non-trained patients.[24,30,32,33,37,39,42,47,51,52]

By way of contrast, the effects of inspiratory muscle training on the distance walked in 6 or 12 min are negligible, and indistinguishable from results in non-trained controls.[17,24,30-32,34,37-39,42,51,54] There was also no change in ability to climb stairs.[31,34,46] The effects of inspiratory muscle training on activities of daily living were variable,[25,31,34,43,46,47,51] and dyspnea tended to be less after inspiratory muscle training.[36,41,43,45,51-54]

Combined regimens

Zack and Palange entered 63 patients with COPD and variable degrees of airflow limitation into a rehabilitation protocol which involved both walking exercise and inspiratory flow-resistive loading.[55] Training lasted 12 weeks.

The level of walking exercise was set to require a level of ventilation that was half-maximal, and training Pbreath was 30 to 50% of PImax. There was a 37% increase in PImax, but the most important finding was that the 12 min walk distance increased by 50 to 70%. Moreover, the percentage of patients improved by 25% or more was the same for those whose FEV$_1$ was low (0.5 to 1.2 litres) as it was for those whose FEV$_1$ was higher (1.2 to 2.5 litres).

Goldstein et al. also studied combined regimens, in an 8 week program.[39]

Half the patients received physical exercise training alone, and half received both inspiratory muscle and physical exercise training. Baseline pulmonary function (FEV$_1$ 33% predicted) and exercise tolerance were the same in both groups. Both groups increased the 6 minute walk distance by 9%, indicating that the increased inspiratory muscle endurance of the inspiratory muscle trained group conferred no advantage to exercise capacity. The negative results of this study might be explained by the observation that both the ventilatory and inspiratory load training stresses may have been lower than those used by Zack and Palange.[55]

Recommendations

Training techniques

Studies of inspiratory muscle training should be extended to patients with diagnoses other than COPD, who are also prone to develop hypercapnic respiratory failure. All studies should include a control population of patients whose diagnosis and degree of impairment is the same as for the study group. In the case of combined interventions, the best controls would be patients who trained with each single regimen alone.

Output variables should be standardized. Specifically, uniform ways of quantifying respiratory muscle endurance should be employed. If possible, more than one way of evaluating respiratory muscle or ventilatory endurance might be used, to facilitate comparison with published data. Standard techniques for evaluating and quantifying dyspnea and activities of daily living should also be incorporated into studies of inspiratory muscle training. Certainly patients should be evaluated for their ability to walk and climb stairs, but it is also useful to quantify their capacity to perform activities requiring the use of the upper extremities.

Exercise and ADL

The concept that the combination of physical exercise and inspiratory loading training would accomplish more than either alone is attractive and deserving of further study. Two aspects of training deserve particular emphasis. First, the level of exercise should be high enough to provide an adequate training stress, probably one that requires minute ventilation during exercise to be 50-60% of maximal. Secondly, the magnitude of the inspiratory load should be enough to make training Pbreath more than 30% of PImax, and the pattern of breathing through the inspiratory load should be regulated to make the inspiratory duty cycle 40-50% of the whole breath duration.

Ventilatory failure

Inspiratory muscle training may well be of value in the prevention or treatment of hypercapnic respiratory failure. Such training might defer the onset of CO$_2$

retention in patients who are so predisposed, and patients with chronic hypercapnia might benefit through stabilization or reduction of $PaCO_2$. During recovery from acute ventilatory failure, the principal benefit of inspiratory muscle training is weaning from mechanical ventilation. To attain these goals, it might well be useful to add interventions which increase diaphragmatic excursion and tidal volume to regimens based on inspiratory loading training.

Final remarks

Effects on respiratory muscles

Interventions designed to displace the diaphragm cephalad and increase its excursion were effective but cumbersome. Breathing exercises which used slow, deep breathing with emphasis on abdominal excursion were about as effective in increasing the excursion of the diaphragm as the head down position and artificial pneumoperitoneum. Moreover, it appears that the degree of airflow limitation in patients who benefited from breathing exercises was similar to that reported in modern studies.

Physical exercise training certainly enhances ventilatory endurance, but generally has little effect on respiratory muscle strength unless the level of exercise is high. Voluntary isocapnic hyperpnea also increases ventilatory endurance, but its effects on respiratory muscle strength and on measures of inspiratory muscle endurance other than maximal sustainable ventilatory capacity are unknown.

Inspiratory loading training increases inspiratory muscle strength, especially if the training stimulus requires Pbreath to be higher then 30% of PImax. Inspiratory loading training also increases the magnitude of the highest tolerable load, and ventilatory endurance for breathing against a high load. It may also be of value in weaning from mechanical ventilation.

Effects on capacity for exercise and ADL

Both voluntary isocapnic hyperpnea and inspiratory resistive loading training increase steady-state bicycle exercise endurance time by more than 60%, but have a negligible effect on 12 minute walk distance. In contrast, physical exercise training programs often increase the 6 or 12 minute walk distance. Only a few studies have carefully examined the effects of training on the capacity for ADL and dyspnea. Most studies report a reduction of dyspnea after training, but this is often based on subjective rather than objective findings.

The most impressive results were obtained when physical exercise and inspiratory load training were combined, and both the ventilatory and the inspiratory load training stresses were appropriately high.

12

References

1. Barach A.L., Beck G.J.: The ventilatory effects of the head-down position in pulmonary emphysema. Am. J. Med. 1954;16:55-60
2. Gayrard P., Becker M., Bergofsky E.H.: The effects of abdominal weights on diaphragmatic position and excursion in man. Clin. Sci. 1968; 35:589-601
3. Gaensler E.A., Carter M.G.: Ventilation measurements in pulmonary emphysema treated with pneumoperitoneum. J. Lab. Clin. Med. 1950; 35:945-959
4. Furman R.H., Callaway J.J.: Artificial pneumoperitoneum in the treatment of pulmonary emphysema. Chest 1950;18:232-243
5. Kory R.C., Roehm D.C., Meneely G.R., Goodwin R.A.: Pulmonary function and circulatory dynamics in artificial pneumoperitoneum. Dis. Chest 1953;23:608-620
6. Callaway J.J., McKusick V.A.: Carbon-dioxide intoxication in emphysema: emergency treatment by artificial pneumoperitoneum. N. Engl. J. Med. 1951; 245:9-13
7. Thoman R.L., Stoker G.L., Ross J.C.: The efficacy of pursed-lips breathing in patients with chronic obstructive pulmonary disease. Am. Rev. Respir. Dis. 1966; 93:100-106
8. Mueller R.E., Petty T.L., Filley G.F.: Ventilation and arterial blood gas changes induced by pursed lips breathing. J. Appl. Physiol. 1970; 28:784-789
9. Miller W.F.: A physiologic evaluation of the effects of diaphragmatic breathing training in patients with chronic pulmonary emphysema. Am. J. Med. 1954; 17:471-484
10. Sinclair J.D.: The effect of breathing exercises in pulmonary emphysema. Thorax 1955; 10:246-249
11. Gimenez M., Uffholtz H., Ferrara G., Plouffe P., Lacoste J.: Exercise training with oxygen supply and directed breathing in patients with chronic airway obstruction. Respiration 1979; 37:157-166
12. Casciari R.J., Fairshter R.D., Harrison A., Morrison J.T., Blackburn C., Wilson A.F.: Effects of breathing retraining in patients with chronic obstructive pulmonary disease. Chest 1981;79:393-398
13. Paul G., Eldridge F., Mitchell J., Fiene T.: Some effects of slowing respiration rate in chronic emphysema and bronchitis. J. Appl. Physiol. 1966; 21:877-882
14. Sergysels R., Willeput R., Lenders D., Vachaudez J.P., Schandevyl W., Hennebert A.: Low frequency breathing at rest and during exercise in severe chronic obstructive bronchitis. Thorax 1979;34:536-539
15. Vandevenne A., Weitzenblum E., Moyses B., Durin M., Rasaholinjanahary J.: Regional lung function changes during abdominal breathing at low frequency and large tidal volume. Bull. Eur. Physiopathol. Respir. 1980; 16:171-184
16. Bellemare F., Grassino A.: Force reserve of the diaphragm in patients with chronic obstructive pulmonary disease. J. Appl. Physiol.: Respir. Environ. Exercise Physiol. 1983;55:8-15
17. Noseda A., Carpiaux J.P., Vandeput W., Prigogine T., Schmerber J.: Resistive inspiratory muscle training and exercise performance in COPD patients. A comparative study with conventional breathing retraining. Bull. Eur. Physiopathol. Respir. 1987; 23:457-463
18. Ioli F., Donner C.F., Fracchia C.: Transdiaphragmatic pressure in the assessment of diaphragmatic and abdominal breathing exercise. Bull. Eur. Physiopathol. Respir. 1982; 18(Suppl.4): 177-180
19. Merrick J., Axen K.: Inspiratory muscle function following abdominal weight exercises in healthy subjects. Physical Therapy 1981; 61:651-656
20. Orenstein D.M., Franklin B.A., Doershuk C.F., Hellerstein H.K., Germann K.J., Horowitz J.G., Stern R.C.: Exercise conditioning and cardiopulmonary fitness in cystic fibrosis: the effects of a three-month supervised running program. Chest 1981;80:392-398
21. Keens T.G., Rrastins I.R.B., Wannamaker E.M., Levison H., Crozier D.N., Bryan A.C.:

Ventilatory muscle endurance training in normal subjects and patients with cystic fibrosis. Am. Rev. Respir. Dis. 1977; 116:853-860

22. Rochester D.F., Goldberg S.K.: Techniques of respiratory physical therapy. Am. Rev. Respir. Dis. 1980;122(5), Part 2:133-146

23. Belman H.J., Kendregan B.A.: Physical training fails to improve ventilatory muscle endurance in patients with chronic obstructive pulmonary disease. Chest 1982;81:440-443

24. Pardy R.L., Rivington R.N., Despas P.J., Macklem P.T.: Inspiratory muscle training compared with physiotherapy in patients with chronic airflow limitation. Am. Rev. Respir. Dis. 1981; 123:421-425

25. Madsen F., Secher N.H., Kay L., Kok-Jensen A., Rube N.: Inspiratory resistance versus general physical training in patients with chronic obstructive pulmonary disease. Eur. J. Respir. Dis. 1985;67:167-176

26. Celli B., Criner G., Rassulo J.: Ventilatory muscle recruitment during unsupported arm exercise in normal subjects. J. Appl. Physiol. 1988; 64:1936-1941

27. Leith D.E., Bradley M.: Ventilatory muscle strength and endurance training. J. Appl. Physiol. 1976;41:508-516

28. Bellemare F.,Grassino A.: Effect of pressure and timing of contraction on human diaphragm fatigue. J. Appl. Physiol. 1982; 53:1190-1195

29. Peress L., McLean P., Woolf C.R., Zamel N.: Ventilatory muscle training in obstructive lung disease. Bull. Eur. Physiopathol. Respir. 1979; 15:91-92

30. Belman M.J., Mittman C.: Ventilatory muscle training improves exercise capacity in chronic obstructive pulmonary disease patients. Am. Rev. Respir. Dis. 1980; 121:273-280

31. Levine S., Weiser P., Gillen J.: Evaluation of a ventilatory muscle endurance training program in the rehabilitation of patients with chronic obstructive pulmonary disease. Am. Rev. Respir. Dis. 1986;133:400-406

32. Ries A.L., Moser K.M.: Comparison of isocapnic hyperventilation and walking exercise training at home in pulmonary rehabilitation. Chest 19086;90:285-289

33. Chen H., Dukes R., Martin B.J.: Inspiratory muscle training in patients with chronic obstructive pulmonary disease. Am. Rev. Respir. Dis. 1985; 131:251-255

34. McKeon J.L., Turner J., Kelly C., Dent A.: The effect of respiratory training on exercise capacity in optimally treated patients with severe chronic airflow limitation. Aust. N.Z. J. Med. 1986; 16:648-652

35. Belman M.J., Shadmehr R.: Targeted resistive ventilatory muscle training in chronic obstructive pulmonary disease. J. Appl. Physiol. 1988; 65:2726-2735

36. Harver A., Mahler D.A., Daubenspeck J.A.: Targeted inspiratory muscle training improves respiratory muscle function and reduces dyspnea in patients with chronic obstructive pulmonary disease. Ann. Int. Med. 1989; 111:117124

37. Larson J.L., Kim M.J., Sharp J.T., Larson D.A.: Inspiratory muscle training with a pressure threshold breathing device in patients with chronic obstructive pulmonary disease. Am. Rev. Respir. Dis. 1988; 138:689-696

38. Flynn M.G., Barter C.D., Nosworthy J.C., Pretto J.J., Rochford P.D., Pierce R.J.: Threshold pressure training, breathing pattern and exercise performance in chronic airflow obstruction. Chest 1989;95:535-540

39. Goldstein R., De Rosie J., Long S., Dolmage T., Avendano M.A.: Applicability of a threshold loading device for inspiratory muscle testing and training in patients with COPD. Chest1989; 96:564-571

40. Belman M.J., Thomas S.G., Lewis M.I.: Resistive breathing training in patients with chronic obstructive pulmonary disease. Chest 1986;90:662-669

14

41. Gross D., Ladd H.W., Riley E.J., Macklem P.T., Grassino A.: The effect of training on strength and endurance of the diaphragm in quadriplegia. Am. J. Med. 1980; 68:27-35
42. Pardy R.L., Rivington R.N., Despas P.J., Macklem P.T.: Effects of inspiratory muscle training on exercise performance in chronic airflow limitation. Am. Rev. Respir. Dis. 1981; 123:426-433
43. Moreno R., Moreno R., Giugliano C., Lisboa C.: Inspiratory muscle training in patients with chronic limitation of airflow. Rev. Med. Chile 1983;111: 647-653
44. Aldrich T.K., Arora N.S., Rochester D.F.: The influence of airway obstruction and respiratory muscle strength on maximal voluntary ventilation in lung disease. Am. Rev. Respir. Dis. 1982; 126:195-199
45. Anderson J.B., Dragsted L., Kann T., Johansen S.H., Nielsen K.B., Karbo E., Bentzen L.: Resistive breathing training in severe chronic obstructive pulmonary disease. Scand. J. Respir. Dis. 1979; 60:151-156
46. Bjerre-Jepsen K., Secher N.H., Kok-Jensen A.: Inspiratory resistance training in severe chronic obstructive pulmonary disease. Eur. J. Respir. Dis. 1981; 62:405-411
47. Sonne L.J., Davis J.A.: Increased exercise performance in patients with severe COPD following inspiratory resistive training. Chest 1982;81:436-439
48. Asher M.I., Pardy R.L., Coates A.L., Thomas E., Macklem P.T.: The effects of inspiratory muscle training in patients with cystic fibrosis. Am. Rev. Respir. Dis. 1982; 126:855-859
49. Belman M.J.: Respiratory failure treated by ventilatory muscle training. Eur. J. Respir. Dis. 1981; 62:391-395
50. Aldrich T.K., Karpel J.P., Uhrlass R.M., Sparapani M.Λ., Eramo D., Ferranti R.: Weaning from mechanical ventilation: adjunctive use of inspiratory muscle resistive training. Crit. Care Med. 1989; 17:143-147
51. Andersen J.B., Falk P.: Clinical experience with inspiratory resistive breathing training. Int. Rehabil. Med. 1984; 6:183-185
52. Falk P., Eriksen A.M., Kolliker K., Andersen J.B.: Relieving dyspnea with an inexpensive and simple method in patients with severe chronic airflow limitation. Eur. J. Respir. Dis. 1985; 66: 181-186
53. Beacham J., Barnes S.M., Walker W., Morse H.B.: Inspiratory resistance training for pulmonary rehabilitation (letter). Chest 1989;96:698-699
54. Jones D.T., Thomson R.A., Sears M.R.: Physical exercise and resistive breathing training in severe chronic airways obstruction - are they effective? Eur. J. Respir. Dis. 1985; 67:159-166
55. Zack M.B., Palange A.V.: Oxygen supplemental exercise of ventilatory and nonventilatory muscles in pulmonary rehabilitation. Chest 1985;88:669-675

2. Rationale for Pulmonary Rehabilitation:Patient Selection

C. F. DONNER, A. BRAGHIROLI, M. LUSUARDI

Division of Pulmonary Disease, Clinica del Lavoro Foundation, Institute of Care and Research, Medical Center of Rehabilitation, Veruno, Italy

Introduction

The benefit of pulmonary rehabilitation is well documented for patients with chronic obstructive pulmonary disease (COPD), whereas there is up to now little evidence[1] or studies in progress[2] about the possible benefits in patients with severe pulmonary impairment who have diagnoses other than COPD.

We will focus on the selection of COPD patients: on the other hand the selection criteria and medications seem appliable to a variety of pulmonary diseases, mostly with restrictive pulmonary function impairment, to be evaluated in the perspective of rehabilitation.

Selection Criteria

There is common agreement that every symptomatic COPD patient should be considered for pulmonary rehabilitation.[3-11]

The selection consequently varies from subjects with mild symptoms and minor abnormalities of spirogram to end stage patients.

Pulmonary rehabilitation is a sort of big container with programs, techniques, tests, devices and drugs which should be picked out and tailored to the very individual problems of each selected patient: probably, the selection of patients should be more properly defined as selection of the program. The evaluator has the task to both conduct a full patient examination and plan a coordinated intervention of his team, using the resources with the aim of returning the patient to the highest performance compatible with his pulmonary handicap.[12,13]

As a director of the program he has the multiple task[14] to:
- assess the patient's willingness to participate in the program
- quantify the required financial resources and check the rules of the third party payers, if any, to avoid further problems of compliance
- analyse the environment and the effective needs of the patient, with the aim of focusing the program on his real expectations
- evaluate the clinical picture, stage the disease, assess its stability and the reasonable margins of improvement. The probationary period to assess the stability of the disease is variable according to the program, and should be particularly careful for patients with indication for long term oxygen and home mechanical ventilation[15,16]
- plan an "ad hoc" program.

Exclusion Criteria

- Patients clinically unstable
- As to cardiac status: recent infarction, congestive heart failure, uncontrolled arrhythmias
- Diseases limiting the rehabilitation: cancer, stroke, organic brain syndromes, hemiplegia
- History of medical noncompliance or loss of motivation: patients who express doubts due to jobs, hobbies, travel plans, etc. should not be admitted.[4-6] Financial problems can obviously be a serious limitation to patients' availability.[12-14]

The admission to intensive programs of patients who continue to smoke is questionable: after the failure of a comprehensive smoking cessation approach, accurate evaluation of future cost-benefit ratio is advisable.

Sometimes a psychological reticence of the patient could be overcome by family support. Family conferences can be usefully organized, a comprehensive information about techniques for domiciliary programs or patients' equipments decreases the anxiety of staying at home.

Family members can be strong motivators or deterrents and even if they refuse a direct involvement in the program it is mandatory to increase their knowledge of the selected plan.

Program Selection

The clinical guidelines often overlap with logistical and behavioral matters and the final choice of the program is usually the sum of various factors. A classification of the different programs is thus very difficult and the only possible subdivision is the location of the subject as an inpatient, outpatient or home care patient.

The most intensive and comprehensive programs are usually reserved for inpatients; home care is usefully applied for long term treatment.[3-11]

Inpatient Programs

Indications
* *Clinical*: Patients limited to two city blocks of slower than normal walking or experiencing breathlessness after almost any exertion have the major benefits. The hospitalization allows performance of diagnostic evaluations (i.e.: hemodynamics, polysomnography, etc.) often necessary to correctly stage the disease and to check its stability, particularly if the medical control at home is considered inadequate.[3-11]
* *Rehabilitative*: It is possible to perform an intensive teaching of rehabilitative techniques or training in the use of new devices and equipments. The exercise and the environment are accurately stated and controlled. The monitoring of the patient is easier.
* *Psychological*: The environment is secure and some particularly anxious patients need a sense of protection at the beginning of the program. Some interventions, such as smoking cessation techniques and dietary changes, can be performed with a greater probability of success if the patient is removed from the daily life situations inducing detrimental habits. Withdrawal from the family can sometimes have a beneficial influence.
* *Organizing*: Transportation can be a problem for old patients and nondrivers. In some countries bad weather conditions can be a major obstacle and an outpatient program could be seriously hindered. These programs are sometimes the only ones reimbursed by third party payers and it is often easier to suspend a job for some days or weeks instead of interrupting it several times per day to follow an outpatient program.

Outpatient Programs

Indications
* *Clinical:* They are usually applied in clinically stable patients, who experience breathlessness only on hills and stairs and can walk indefinitely at their own pace.[3-11]
* *Rehabilitative:* They can be the completion of an inpatient program and are used to reinforce continuity in the application of exercises, maneuvres, use of equipments after hospital discharge.
* *Psychological*: The home environment is maintained: this is important in children and elderly patients who suffer in being hospitalized. The family is more involved and can reinforce the compliance of the patient.

18

* *Organizing:* There should not be transportation problems and the program must not interfere with the job.

Home Care Programs

Indications
* *Clinical:* Patients who need long term treatments usually have the greatest benefits, especially the so called "revolving door" patients, with repeated hospitalizations. End stage terminal patients who want to stay at home and anxious and confused subjects take advantage of this kind of assistance.[17]
* *Rehabilitative:* Long term oxygen therapy and home mechanical ventilation are applied indefinitely in patients who require close supervision and a specific knowledge of technical and clinical problems.[18] Patients who require a period of follow up after an inpatient program can be usefully included.[17]
* *Organizing:* The original concept of assistance is reversed by these programs: the hospital meets the patient instead of the patient going to hospital. An effective home care organization is not easy to develop as it requires a considerable investment at the beginning, with specialized team and resources. The lowering of health costs, with a dramatic decrease in the number of days spent in hospital, and the substantial improvement in patient care usually repays the initial effort when a sufficient number of patients is taken in charge.[19,20]

In conclusion we can underline that only a careful assessment of a wide variety of components can lead to a correct selection of the most suitable rehabilitation program for the individual patient. An adequate balance between clinical picture and psycho-social and environmental needs should characterize a well tailored plan of treatment inducing greater patient motivation and stronger family support.

References

1. Foster S., Thomas III H.M.: Pulmonary rehabilitation in lung disease other than chronic obstructive pulmonary disease. Am. Rev. Respir. Dis. 1990; 141:601-604
2. Donner C.F., Braghiroli A., Ioli F., Zaccaria S.: Long-term oxygen therapy in patients with diagnoses other than COPD. Lung 1990; Suppl:776-781
3. American Thoracic Society: Guidelines for pulmonary rehabilitation. Am. Rev. Respir. Dis. 1981; 124:663-666
4. American Thoracic Society: Standards for the diagnosis and care of patients with obstructive pulmonary disease (COPD) and asthma. Am. Rev. Respir. Dis. 1987; 136:225-244
5. Maddox S.E., Selecky P.A., Barry M.S., McLean D.L.: Organization and structure of a pulmonary rehabilitation program. In: Hodgkin J.E., Zorn E.G., Connors G.L. (Eds.):*Pulmonary Rehabilitation. Guidelines to Success* Boston: Butterworth Publishers, 1984; 9-22
6. Woolf C.R.: Respiratory Rehabilitation: a Practical Guide. Toronto, Tower Liths Company Ltd, 1986; 28-29

7. Hodgkin J.E.: Pulmonary rehabilitation: structure, components and benefits. J. Cardiopulmonary Rehabil. 1988;11:423-434
8. Petty T.L.: Pulmonary Rehabilitation Basics of RD. New York, American Thoracic Society, 1975
9. Hudson L.D., Pierson D.J.. Comprehensive respiratory care for patients with chronic obstructive pulmonary disease. Medical Clinics of North America 1981; 65:629-645
10. Lertzman M.M., Cherniak R.M.. Rehabilitation of patients with chronic obstructive pulmonary disease. Am. Rev. Respir. Dis. 1976; 114:1145-1165
11. Hodgkin J.E., Zorn E.G., Connors G.L.: Pulmonary rehabilitation: definition and essential components. In: Hodgkin J.E., Zorn E.G., Connors G.L. (Eds.):*Pulmonary Rehabilitation. Guidelines to Success* Boston: Butterworth Publishers, 1984, 1-7
12. Yee A.R., Hodgkin J.E.: The role of the medical director. In: Hodgkin J.E., Zorn E.G., Connors G.L. (Eds.):*Pulmonary Rehabilitation. Guidelines to Success* Boston: Butterworth Publishers, 1984, 22-23
13. Connors G.A., Hodgkin J.E., Asmus R.M.: A careful assessment is crucial to successful pulmonary rehabilitation. J. Cardiopulmonary Rehabil. 1988; 11:435-438
14. Hodge-Hilton T., Herrmann D.W., Hills R.L., Feenstra L. Archibald C. :Initial evaluation of the pulmonary rehabilitation candidate. In: Hodgkin J.E., Zorn E.G., Connors G.L. (Eds.):*Pulmonary Rehabilitation. Guidelines to Success* Boston: Butterworth Publishers, 1984, 27-44
15. SEP TASK GROUP LTO: Recommendations for long term oxygen. Eur. Respir. J. 1989; 2:160-164
16. Levi-Valensi P., Weitzenblum E., Pedinielli J.L., Racineux J.L., Duwoos H.: Three months follow up of arterial blood gas determination in candidates for long term oxygentherapy. Am. Rev. Respir. Dis. 1986;133:547-551
17. Meany-Handy J., Lareau S.C.: The role of home care. In: Hodgkin J.E., Zorn E.G., Connors G.L. (Eds.):*Pulmonary Rehabilitation. Guidelines to Success* Boston: Butterworth Publishers, 1984, 311-322
18. Hill N.S.: Home care of ventilator-assisted and ventilator-dependent patients. J. Cardiopulmonary Rehabil. 1988; 11:462-472
19. Schneider E.L.: Options to control the rising health care costs of older Americans. JAMA 1989; 261:907-908
20. Council on Scientific Affairs: Home care in the 1990s. JAMA 1990; 263:1241-1244

3. The Goals of Pulmonary Rehabilitation

H.FOLGERING, R.DEKHUIJZEN, N.COX, C.VAN HERWAARDEN

Department of Pulmonary Diseases, Dekkerswald Medical Center, University of Nijmegen, The Netherlands

Introduction

Patients with pulmonary diseases tend to get caught in a vicious circle. The disease causes dyspnea, especially during physical activities. Consequently these activities will be negatively rewarded, and the patient may eventually be conditioned not to undertake any activities at all. This will lead to inactivity, frustrations and social isolation.[2]

The inactivity in itself will be the cause of a reduced physical fitness, and further activities will be even more difficult.[3]

Pulmonary rehabilitation can break this circle at various locations: it partially reduces the impaired lung function by an improved patient-compliance to proper medication, it reduces the number and intensity of the complaints, it gives the patient a greater insight in the underlying pathophysiology of the disease, and it will improve the fitness of the patient.

The psychological effect of a rehabilitation treatment results in a considerable improvement of the patient's self-esteem, decrease of depression, and improves the feelings of inadequacy.

Definitions

Pulmonary rehabilitation is defined as an art of medical practice in which an individually tailored, multidisciplinary program is formulated. It is indicated for patients suffering from complex problems in relation to their pulmonary disease.

The goals of pulmonary rehabilitation are:

1. A decrease of physical and psychological manifestations of the underlying disease, i.e. a reduction of the *impairment* due to the disease.
2. An increase in physical and mental fitness and performance, reduction of the *disability*.
3. A maximal social reintegration of the patient, thus lowering of the *handicap*.

The ultimate goal is a maximal functional capacity, allowed by the pulmonary disturbance and overall situation.

According to the WHO-classifications, the impairment is the damage due to the disease at the level of the organ; the disability describes the manifestation of the disease in the physical and psychological performance of the patient; and the handicap implies the social or vocational set back of the patient due to the disease.

The methods by which these goals may be achieved are used in a program, tailored to each individual patient. It consists of:

a. An accurate diagnosis of the disease and of the functional limitations of the patient.
b. Education about the disease, its pathophysiology, the use of medication, the use of a peak flow meter, and the avoidance of harmful or aggravating stimuli, e.g. *smoking*.
c. Physical training to improve the physical fitness and performance,
d. Psychosocial support.[4]

The program should be based on an adequate diagnosis of the extent and character of the limitations of the individual patient.

Limiting Factors for Physical Performance

During exercise the metabolism in the working muscles is increased; more oxygen has to be transported to these muscles, and more carbon dioxide has to be eliminated. The various physiological systems involved in this gas transport chain, and their interaction, are shown in the model of a power plant in figure 1.

The coal for the power plant (oxygen) is taken up from the external environment by a crane (the lungs) and loaded into a funnel.

After unloading the oxygen, the crane has to pick up the ashes (CO_2) from a bunker with a narrow opening (airways). When the opening of the bunker is further narrowed (bronchial obstruction), and when the crane has to work very hard, the level of the ashes in the bunker will rise (hypercapnia).

The coal in the funnel will fall on the conveyer belt; its flow is limited by the width of the opening of the funnel (diffusion capacity of the alveolar-capillary membrane). The position of the funnel above the conveyer belt models the

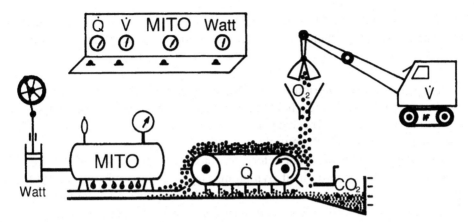

Fig. 1. A model of the mechanisms of gas transport from the ambient air to the mitochondria and *vice versa*.

ventilation-perfusion matching. The transport of the oxygen by the circulation is represented by the conveyer belt. The compartments on the belt are equivalent to the hemoglobin; the extent to which the compartments are filled represents the saturation of the hemoglobin with oxygen.

The speed of the belt (cardiac output) determines the delivery of the oxygen to the place where the actual combustion takes place: in the mitochondria of the working muscles. Not all oxygen is extracted in the muscles, but some is 'spilled' into the venous system. The underside of the conveyer belt sweeps the ashes (CO_2) to the bunker, from where they are removed by the crane. Malfunctioning of the steam engine occurs in enzymatic deficiencies at the mitochondrial level. Somewhere in the powerplant there is a control room (central nervous system) where information about the functioning of the crane, the conveyer belt, the steam engine, and of the power output, converge. The controller in this control room interprets these incoming signals and may decide (correctly or incorrectly) that one or more machines in the plant are overloaded, and therefore he may decide to limit the output of the plant.

The output of the power plant is limited by the slowest subunit in the plant. In normal subjects this limitation comes from the conveyor belt. In patients the limitations may come from other subunits in the powerplant.

Maximal Exercise Testing

In order to test the working capacity and the limiting factors of a pulmonary patient, a maximal exercise test has to be performed. Measurement of arterial blood gas values, heart rate and blood pressure, pleural pressures, and ventilatory and oxygen consumption parameters, will provide essential information about the gas transport in the patient. An incremental test, lasting approximately 10 minutes, is quite useful for assessment of the maximal working capacity, and the limiting factors.

The physiological criterion for true maximal exercise or work performance is fulfilled when the patient reaches the maximal capacity of one of the components of the total gas transport mechanism: the lungs, the heart and circulation, or the (enzymatic) processes in the muscles.[5,6]

Apart from the physiological criteria for maximal exercise, very often a symptom limited maximum is defined. Symptoms may originate from proprioceptors in the working muscles, in joints, in those parts of the body that are in contact with the ergometry apparatus, from temperature sensors, from receptors in airways, from respiratory muscles, etc.[7] The incoming signals from these receptors are processed and interpreted in the central nervous system, depending on the patient's mood, previous experiences, personality factors etc. Therefore "symptom limited" maximal tests are difficult to measure and to interpret. The individual interpretation of these symptoms may change considerably during a rehabilitation program.

In the context of the assessment of fitness or work-capacity of patients with pulmonary diseases, an ergometric exercise test should be truely maximal in the physiological sense, under optimal bronchodilatory treatment. Submaximal tests are often used in normal subjects; the relationship between heart rate and external work load (or oxygen consumption) is then extrapolated to the point of the age-specific maximal heart rate (cardiocirculatory limitation). From this point the maximal oxygen consumption is calculated.[6] It is clear that in patients who are not limited by their heart and circulation (conveyer belt in the model), this kind of indirect determination of the maximal work load cannot be applied. Exercise testing in these patients will have to be continued until one of the gas transport systems reaches its maximum. Only maximal tests will show where the limitation of the individual patient is located; this will have important consequences for the ensuing rehabilitation treatment.[8]

Several categories of patients can be distinguished on the basis of their type of exercise limitation:

Cardiocirculatory Limitation

Patients with light to moderate asthma or COPD show this type of exercise limitation, as in normal subjects. The impairment of these patients consists of a minor airway obstruction, usually with FEV_1-values above approximately 1.5 liter, or above 60% of the reference value.[14]

In an incremental exercise test these patients, like normal subjects, continue until they reach their age-specific maximal heart rate, or until they produce approximately 10 mmol/liter of lactate. At maximal exercise they still have a considerable breathing reserve.[5] The latter is defined as the difference between the maximal breathing capacity (MBC)[10] and the actual ventilation (MBC can be measured spirometrically, or calculated by 37.5 x FEV_1). This breathing reserve at maximal work load in mildly obstructed patients can also be inferred from arterial PCO_2-values, which are lower than the resting values. Apparently the ventilatory system is capable of "blowing off" more CO_2 than the body produces during maximal exercise. However, the circulatory system cannot transport sufficient O_2 to the working muscles. These have to switch over to an anaerobic metabolism, resulting in lactic acid production.

This kind of patient is not limited by the impairment of his/her pulmonary disease; usually they only "suffer" from poor physical fitness.[15] In a rehabilitation program they can participate in endurance training. A training program with exercise levels above 50% of the maximal aerobic power, or 75-85% of the maximal heart rate, is necessary for achieving an improved fitness. In such endurance training sessions, the level of exercise remains below the ones that cause lactate accumulation. They should be undertaken at least 3 times a week, for at least half an hour.[6] With such a training program, it is possible to attain levels of fitness which often allow the patients to return to work. The number of days spent on sick-leave can be reduced substantially.

In a controlled study on 44 patients with mild obstructive lung disease (mean FEV_1 68% pred), Cox[16] has shown that a 3-month program (38 hrs/week) can substantially improve the exercise performance on the bicycle ergometer, the 12 min walking distance, and the subjective feeling of well-being.

They can cope substantially better with their disease. The number of visits to their general practitioners, or to their chest physicians, in the years after such a rehabilitation program, is substantially reduced, as well as the number of hospital admissions[3,16,17] (Tab. I)

These effects remain for at least two years. It is essential that the patients should continue the training after the end of the actual rehabilitation program. Inactivity will eliminate the effects of the rehabilitation program within a matter of weeks. Advising the patients to join a sports or physical fitness club can provide them with a social support, and may help him/her to carry out the good intentions made during the rehabilitation treatment. Their habits in participating in sports or physical exercise can also be changed considerably (Tab. I).

Ventilatory Limitation

In this group of patients, the crane of the powerplant cannot cope with the rate of production of ashes (CO_2). These patients with chronic obstructive pulmonary disease usually have approximate FEV_1-values below 1.5 liter or below 60% of

Table I. Changes in 44 patients with cardiocirculatory limitation, due to a 3 months pulmonary rehabilitation program.[16]

	Before	3 Months	12 Months	24 Months
VO$_2$ max	2.18±0.03	2.56±0.05***	2.34±0.04*	2.37±0.05*
12 MWD (m)	1639±38	2139±44***	1958±44**	1925±60**
Cycling ±	2.3±0.1	2.8±0.1***	2.9±0.2*	2.8±0.1*
Well-being	21.0±1.1	30.1±1.4***	26.0±1.3	27.1±1.2*
Visits GP °	3.7±0.4		1.8±0.5	1.4±0.5
Hospit Days x	9.1±1.7		5.7±1.6	0.1±1.7*
Workdays/wk	2.1±0.4			2.4±0.4*

Values are means + SEM.
*: p=0.05 **: p=0.01 ***: p=0.001 significance of changes versus value before, corrected for changes in control group (ANOVA).
+ : cycling habits scored as 1=never; 2=sometimes; 3=frequently; 4=often.
°: number of visits per year to the general practitioner.
x: number of days (per year) admitted to a hospital for pulmonary problems.
VO$_2$max: maximal oxygen consumption (l/min).
12MWD: Twelve minute walking distance (meters).
3 Months: at end of rehabilitation period.
12 and 24 Months: 12 and 24 months respectively, after start of rehabilitation program.

predicted. At maximal exercise the breathing reserve (MBC minus actual minute ventilation) is zero or even negative. The final criterion for ventilatory limitation is an increased arterial PCO$_2$-value. Since the CO$_2$ elimination is limited by the alveolar ventilation, hypercapnia is the essential indicator that this part of the transport mechanism cannot cope with the metabolic needs of the body during exercise.[5]

If ventilation is insufficient for eliminating the produced CO$_2$, then it should also be insufficient for an adequate intake of oxygen. However, not every ventilatory-limited patient becomes hypoxemic during hypercapnic exercise. Many of these patients have a ventilation/perfusion mismatch at resting conditions, resulting in lowered arterial PO$_2$ levels. During exercise, ventilation and cardiac output both increase, and the matching of the two may also improve.[18] This improved ventilation/perfusion matching will counteract the effects of the relative hypoventilation on the arterial PO$_2$. The arterial PO$_2$ levels during exercise in many of these ventilatory-limited patients may therefore remain unchanged as compared to the resting values.

The ventilatory limitation is a result of an imbalance between the ventilatory load of moving sufficient air through the obstructed airways and the working capacity of the respiratory muscles. Respiratory muscle function can also be impaired in these patients, because of the position of the diaphragm on its length-tension curve due to hyperinflation, and because of the deconditioning of the muscles due to relative inactivity. The function of these muscles can be assessed by measuring pleural (esophageal) pressures before and during the maximal exercise test.[20]

Before the ergometry starts, the patient is asked to perform maximal dynamic inspiratory and expiratory maneuvers against a (semi-) closed airway. The measurement of maximal inspiratory and expiratory pressures (Pi max and Pe max) in this context should be made in a dynamic situation. In our hands, the procedure of a maximal sniff for measurement of Pi max, as proposed by Koulouris et al.,[20] appeared to be very adequate, and easy to perform by the patients. For the Pe max the patient is asked to cough, or make a short Valsalva maneuver.

These forces are usually lower than in normal subjects. During an incremental exercise test, the amplitude of the inspiratory and expiratory pleural pressure swings increases. Normal subjects will show negative pleural pressures during the whole respiratory cycle, at rest and during exercise. Only at maximal work load, the expiratory pressures will become slightly positive, indicating an active expiration. Patients with moderate to severe airway obstruction, or with a reduced elastic recoil of the lung parenchyma, show positive expiratory pleural pressures, sometimes at rest, always in the early stages of exercise (Fig 2). Presumably, active expiration contributes to the sensation of dyspnea, and makes the patient stop exercising. At maximal exercise, the pleural pressures may equal the maximal pressures generated before the exercise test. This indicates exercise limitation due to respiratory muscle failure, and consequently is a good indication for inspiratory muscle training.[14]

Recording the pleural pressure swings also provides the opportunity to quantify the inspiratory work load by calculating a parameter like the Time-Tension Index (TTI) at rest and at various stages of exercise.

This index calculates the actual inspiratory pressure (Pi act) relative to the maximal attainable inspiratory pressure (Pi max), multiplied by the duration of the inspiration (Ti) relative to the duration of the total respiratory cycle (Ttot).

$$TTI = (Pi\ act/Pi\ max) \times (Ti/Ttot)$$

A TTI-value of approximately 0.15 for transdiaphragmatic pressures has been used as an indication for fatigue of that muscle.[21]

Dyspnea, caused by hypercapnia, increased respiratory muscle load, positive expiratory pleural pressures, or by a combination of these factors, is usually the reason for the patients to stop exercising.

Pulmonary rehabilitation of these ventilatory-limited patients is aimed at ergonomics: increasing the efficiency of the human "machine" by improving the performance at the same level of oxygen consumption. Calisthenics,[23] interval training and mobilization exercises also help in this respect. Furthermore breathing

28

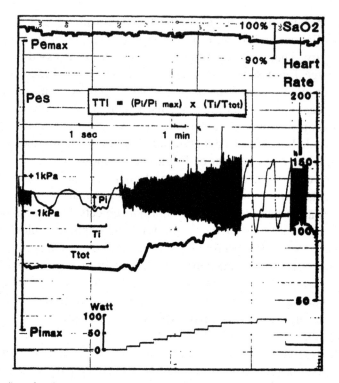

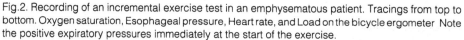

Fig.2. Recording of an incremental exercise test in an emphysematous patient. Tracings from top to bottom. Oxygen saturation, Esophageal pressure, Heart rate, and Load on the bicycle ergometer Note the positive expiratory pressures immediately at the start of the exercise.

retraining that emphasizes a low respiratory frequency will improve gas exchange and reduce dead space ventilation.[24]

If the pre-rehabilitation ergometry has shown a high respiratory muscle load or even failure, inspiratory muscle training will be beneficial, since it will improve Pi max.

Dekhuijzen[25] studied 40 COPD-patients with a mean FEV_1 of 1.48 liter (48% ref. value) and a ventilatory limitation to exercise. All patients received a 10-week pulmonary rehabilitation program; twenty of them received additional target-flow inspiratory muscle training. With this training, inspiratory flow, inspiratory resistance, and timing (Ti and Te), are imposed in such a way that 70% of Pi max is generated at every inspiration. Thus the workload for the inspiratory muscles during the training is well defined.

The group of patients that received additional inspiratory muscle training showed significantly more improvement of the 12 minute walking distance than the group who did not receive this training (Table II). A control group who received only inspiratory muscle training without a rehabilitation treatment did not improve at all. This is in agreement with findings of other investigators.[26]

Table II. Results of a 10 week pulmonary rehabilitation program in 40 patients with a ventilatory limitation, and additional target flow inspiratory muscle training in 20 of them.[25]

	Before	10 Weeks	12 Months
VO$_2$ max			
PR	1.46±0.5	1.62±0.6	1.50±0.5
PR±IMT	1.37±0.5	1.47±0.6*	1.49±0.5
12 MWD			
PR	1057±284	1251±354**	1222±321**
PR±IMT	1046±323	1309±376 **°	1262±368**
ADL scores			
PR	6.3±2.3	7.7±2.3	7.4±2.4
PR±MT	6.2±2.4	8.4±2.2	7.0±2.4

Values are means and standard deviations.
VO$_2$ max (l/min); 12 MWD = twelve minutes walking distance (meters);
ADL = activities of daily life (points scored on questionnaire; possible scores ranging from 0 to 11);
PR = pulmonary rehabilitation;
IMT = Inspiratory Muscle Training;
** = $p < 0.01$ data compared to value before PR;
° = $p < 0.05$ PR *versus* PR+IMT (Mann Whitney U-test).

The patients should be coached and supervised during the initial inspiratory muscle training sessions, by a physiotherapist. Adequate inspiratory muscle training will improve the strength and endurance of the respiratory muscles.[27]

It is also possible that adaptation to the sensation of dyspnea occurs as a beneficial side-effect.

In very severely ventilatory-limited patients, the respiratory muscles may be overloaded even when performing the activities of daily life. These muscles need complete rest before they are able to continue their work, even when the patient is at rest.[28] Various methods of mechanical ventilation at home are still under investigation. The results are conflicting and are difficult to interpret.

Oxygen-uptake Limitation

In patients with pulmonary emphysema or with interstitial pulmonary diseases, the gas transport of oxygen during exercise (increased oxygen consumption) is limited at the level of the alveolar-capillary membrane. In the powerplant model, the opening of the funnel is too narrow. In emphysematous patients the total surface

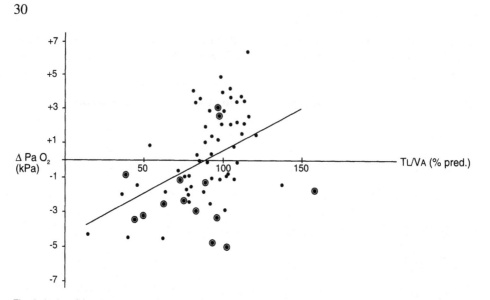

Fig. 3. A plot of the change in PaO_2 at maximal exercise, *versus* the value of TLCO for carbon monoxide (% ref value). The dots are from patients with an obstructive pulmonary disease; the solid circles are from patients with interstitial lung disease. The TLCO-value appears to be a very bad predictor of exercise changes in PaO_2.

of the membrane is reduced and therefore the pulmonary capillary volume is also reduced. Measuring the diffusing capacity with carbon monoxide (TLCO) will not predict exercise hypoxia in the individual patient (Fig. 3). Measurement of arterial oxygen saturation with a pulse oxymeter during the exercise testing provides continuous information about the hypoxemia during the exercise test. An arterial oxygen desaturation below approximately 80% is one of the few reasons for stopping an exercise test by the supervising doctor.

An oxygen-uptake limitation often is concomitant with a ventilatory limitation and alveolar hypoventilation. In order to differentiate between the various possible causes of hypoxemia, it can be helpful to calculate the alveolar to arterial oxygen difference ($AaDO_2$). This difference also increases in normal subjects.[5,20] When the $AaDO_2$ increases by more than 2 kPa (15 mmHg) from rest to maximal exercise, it is reasonable to assume that the oxygen uptake is impaired at the level of the alveolar-capillary membrane, either by a diffusion problem or by shunting.

It is not clear why these patients stop exercising. Usually they stop before the hypoxemia is so severe that the hypoxic ventilatory drive contributes substantially to the sensation of dyspnea.

Another factor may be the mechanics of breathing. In emphysematous patients as well as in patients with interstitial lung diseases, the work of breathing is increased.[23] This will contribute to dyspnea. Furthermore, the working muscles of these patients usually are in a state of detraining. This means that the capillary density in the muscles and the amount and size of the mitochondria in the muscle fibers is reduced. In the model, the left end of the conveyer belt is not close enough to the boiler, or there are not enough burning places in the furnace. Much lactate is therefore produced locally, and will be eliminated rather slowly, because of the low capillary density. Finally, if the cardiac function of these patients is impaired, exercise may lead to overfilling of the pulmonary circulation: a potent stimulus to dyspnea.

Rehabilitation of these patients should contain ergonomics: the objective being the increased efficiency of the human machine, and increased ratio of external work load over oxygen consumption. Breathing exercises aimed at low-frequency breathing will keep the dead space ventilation relatively low. For many patients additional oxygen is necessary to remain normoxic during exercise, and thus to allow them to increase their performance.[29,30,31,32] Exercising with additional oxygen improves the exercise performance in the acute situation. In the long run it also may improve the condition of the peripheral muscles by increasing the capillary density and the amount and size of the mitochondria. This allows better peripheral oxygen extraction, and thus a better usage of the limited amount of oxygen available to the patients with impaired lungs.

The amount of oxygen needed to keep the patients normoxic during exercise can be titrated in an exercise test with on-line monitoring of the arterial oxygen saturation with a pulse oxymeter. In our experience, nasal prongs are usually not adequate for sufficient oxygen administration during exercise. A venturimask, or intratracheal administration of oxygen, is more efficient for these patients.

Psychophysiological Limitations

When a patient stops an exercise test without reaching the maximal capacity of one of the physiological gas transport mechanisms, i.e. no maximal heart rate, hypercapnia, hypoxemia, significant metabolic acidosis, or maximal esophageal pressures, then it can be assumed that the reasons for stopping are psychogenic. Timed walking tests are also determined by psychological factors, as well as by spirometric parameters.[33] There are several psychophysiological reasons: perception of dyspnea, anticipation of dyspnea, and even exercise phobia. Psychosocial aspects may also play a role: the attitude that a person with a pulmonary disease is a patient, and should therefore not exert him- or herself. This patient-behavior is either self-imposed or imposed by the family and other well-meaning bystanders.[2]

In patients with bronchial hyperreactivity the stimulation of irritant receptors in the airways may lead to exercise-induced bronchoconstriction, and/or to hyperventilation. The exercise-induced bronchoconstriction usually can be treated adequately with bronchodilators, and is very seldom a reason for nonparticipation in exercise or sports.

Hyperventilation occurs especially in psychologically stressing situations, and after stopping exercising. There is an afterdischarge phenomenon in the respiratory centers in the brainstem as described by Eldridge et al.[34]: once the neuronal activity in the brainstem is increased, e.g. due to exercise, it cannot abruptly return to its resting level, but it decays slowly with a certain time-constant. This hyperventilation causes hypocapnia, and subsequently frightening symptoms such as dizziness, palpitations, paresthesiae, faintness, and sometimes chest pain.

If such disquieting symptoms regularly happen after exercising, the patient will become conditioned not to exercise in order to prevent them from occurring. Therapeutic interventions with hyperventilation problems should mainly be aimed at changing the cognitions about the body sensations.

In terms of the power plant model: the man in the control room has to be

Table III. Flowchart on interpretation of maximal exercise tests and the ensuing consequences for the rehabilitation treatment.

Maximal exercise test		Diagnosis		Therapy
$Hr >= 220 - age$ and/or $BE > 10$ mmol/l	→ yes →	cardiocircul limitation	→	endurance training
↓ no ↓				
$PaCO_2$ max > $PaCO_2$ rest and $PaCO_2$ max > 5.5kPa	→ yes →	ventilatory limitation	→	calisthenics ergonomics interval training
↓ no ↓				
$Pes >= Ples$ max or $Pes >= PEes$ max or $TTI > 15$	→ yes →	ventil. muscle failure	→	ergonomics inspir. muscle training breathing exercise
↓ no ↓				
PaO_2 max < PaO_2 rest and $\Delta(A-a)DO_2$ 2 kPa	→ yes →	diff- perfusion limitation	→	calisthenics ADL training ergonomics supplemental O_2
↓ no ↓				
exercise test was not maximal	→ yes →	psychogenic limitation	→	education endurance training self confidence

reeducated about reading the meters, and about taking (not) actions at high readings of these meters.

The rehabilitation program will recondition the patient, by reestablishing selfconfidence, and by teaching breathing patterns with low respiratory frequencies.

Conclusions

An accurate diagnosis is the beginning of all rehabilitation. Lung function tests will give an indication about the physical aspects of the impairment caused by the disease.

Adequate pharmacological treatment until maximal lung function parameters are obtained is a prerequisite before starting the actual rehabilitation program. True maximal exercise testing, according to physiological criteria, is essential in evaluating what the patient can perform, and thus the extent of the physical aspects of the disability.

Furthermore the maximal exercise test will identify limiting factors in the gas transport chain. Rehabilitation should aim especially at improving the function of this limiting factor.

Table III shows a flow-chart about the interpretation of the maximal exercise test, and the conclusions to be made from this test. Psychological support, improving the performance of the patient, changing negative attitudes towards the disease and towards the patient's concepts of what is realistically possible in spite of the disease, will lower the handicap by improving the social functioning of the patient, and by reducing his/her disadvantages as compared to normal people, at home or at work.

This study was partly supported by the Netherland's Asthma Foundation.

References

1. American Thoracic Society: Standards for the diagnosis and care of patients with chronic obstructive pulmonary disease (COPD) and asthma. Am. Rev. Respir. Dis. 1987; 136: 225-244
2. Sandhu H.S.: Psychosocial issues in chronic obstructive pulmonary disease. Clinics in Chest Medicine 1986; 7: 629-642
3. Belman M.J.: Exercise in chronic obstructive pulmonary disease. Clinics in Chest Medicine 1986; 7: 585-597
4. American Thoracic Society.: Pulmonary rehabilitation Am. Rev. Respir. Dis. 1981; 124: 663-666
5. Wassermann K., Hansen J.E., Sue D.Y., Whipp B.J.: *Principles of Exercise Testing and Interpretation*. Philadelphia, Lea & Febiger 1987
6. Astrand P.O., Rodahl K.: *Textbook of work physiolgy*. New York, McGraw-Hill 1977
7. Altose M.D., Chonan T.,Cherniak N.S.: Respiratory sensations during exercise, hypercapnia and voluntary hyperventilation. In: C.v.Euler & M.KatzSalomon (eds.) *Respiratory Psychophysiology*. London, MacMillan Press 1988; 79-86

34

8. Wasserman K., Sue D.Y., Casaburi R., Moricca R.B.: Selection criteria for exercise training in pulmonary rehabilitation. Eur. Respir. J. 1989; 2: suppl 7, 604S-610S

9. Scherer D., Kaltenbach M.: Häufigkeit lebensberohlicher Komplikationen beider ergometrischen Belastungsuntersuchungen. Dtsch. Med. Wschr. 1979; 104: 1161-1166

10. Jones N.L., Campbell E.L.M.: *Clinical Exercise Testing.* Philadelphia, WB Saunders, 1982

11. Yeh M.P., Gardner R.M., Adams T.D., Yanowitz F.G., Crapo R.O.: "Anaerobic threshold": problems of determination and validation. J. Appl. Physiol. 1983,55,1178-1186

12. Hagberg J.M., Coyle J.E., Carroll J.M., Miller W., Martin H., Brooke M.H.: Exercise hyperventilation in patients with McArdle's disease. J. Appl. Physiol. 1982; 52: 991-994

13. Casaburi R., Wasserman K., Patessio A., Loli F., Zanaboni S., Donner CF.: A new perspective in pulmonary rehabilitation: an anaerobic threshold as a discriminant in training. Eur. Respir. J. 1989; 2: suppl 2, 618S-623S

14. Dekhuizen P., Folgering H., Herwaarden C. van.: Target-flow inspiratory muscle training and pulmonary rehabilitation in ventilatory limited patients. Eur. Respir. J. 1989; 2: suppl 8, 791S

15. Clark C.J., Cochrame L.M.: Assessment of work performance in asthma for determination of cardiorespiratory fitness and training capacity. Thorax 1988; 43: 745-749

16. Cox N.J.M.: *Effects of a pulmonary rehabilitation programme in patients with obstructive lung diseases.* Thesis, University of Nijmegen (The Netherlands), 1990

17. Cox N.J.M., Herwaarden C.L.A. van, Folgering H., Binkhorst R.A.: Exercise and training in patients with chronic obstructive lung disease. Sports Medicine 1988; 6: 180-192

18. Thews G., Meyer D.: Der pulmonale Gasaustausch bei körperlicher Belastung. Atemwege Lungenkrankh. 1987; 13: 271 -277

19. Bye P.T.P., Farkas G.A., Roussos Ch.: Respiratory factors limiting exercise. Ann. Rev. Physiol. 1983; 45: 439-451

20. Koulouris N., Mulvey D.A., Laroche C.M., Sawicka E.H., Green M., Moxham J.:The measurement of inspiratory muscle strength by sniff esophageal, nasopharyngeal, and mouth pressures. Am. Rev. Respir. Dis. 1989; 139: 641-646

21. Bellamare F., Grassino A.: Effect of pressure and timing of contraction on human diaphragmatic fatigue. J. Appl. Physiol. 1982; 53: 1190-1195

22. Freedman S., Cooke N.T., Moxham J.: Production of lactic acid by respiratory muscles. Thorax 1983; 38: 50-54

23. Gimenez M.: Exercise training in patients with chronic airways obstruction. Eur. Respir. J. 1989; 2: suppl 7,611S-617S

24. Meerhaeghe A. van, Sergysels R.: Control of breathing during exercise in patients with chronic airflow limitation with or without hypercapnia. Chest 1983; 84: 565-570

25. Dekhuijzen P.N.R.: *Target-flow inspiratory muscle training and pulmonary rehabilitation in patients with chronic obstructive pulmonary disease.* Thesis University of Nijmegen (The Netherlands), 1989

26. Grassino A.: Inspiratory muscle training in COPD patients. Eur. Respir. J. 1989; 2: suppl 7, 581 S-586S

27. Levine S., Weiser P., Gillen J.: Evaluation of a ventilatory muscle endurance training program in the rehabilitation of patients with chronic obstructive pulmonary disease. Am. Rev. Respir. Dis. 1986; 133: 400-406

28. Green M.: Respiratory muscle rest. Eur. Respir. J. 1989; 2: suppl 7, 578S-580S

29. Jones N.L., Jones G., Edwards R.H.T.: Exercise tolerance in chronic airway obstruction Am.Rev.Respir. Dis. 1971; 103: 477-491

30. Light R.W., Mahutte C.K., Stansbury D.W., Fisher C.E., Brown S.E.: Relationship between improvement in exercise performance with supplemental oxygen and hypoxic ventilatory drive in patients with chronic airflow obstruction. Chest 1989; 95: 751-756
31. Davidson A.C., Leach R., George R.J.D., Geddes D.M.: Supplemental oxygen and exercise ability in chronic obstructive airway disease. Thorax 1988; 43: 965-971
32. Stein D.A., Bradley B.L., Miller W.C.: Mechanisms of oxygen effects on exercise in patients with chronic obstructive pulmonary disease. Chest 1982; 81: 6-10
33. Jones P.W., Baveystok C.M., Littlejohns P.: Anxiety, depression, walking speed and spirometry in chronic airways obstruction. Thorax 1988; 43: 858P
34. Eldridge F.L., Gill-Kumar P.: Central neural respiratory drive and afterdischarge. Respir. Physiol. 1980; 40: 49-63

4. Economic Evaluation in Chronic Obstructive Pulmonary Disease

R.S. GOLDSTEIN, E.H. GORT

West Park Hospital, Mount Sinai Hospital, Department of Medicine, University of Toronto, Ontario, Canada

Introduction

Respiratory rehabilitation programs are widely accepted as important in the management of patients with chronic obstructive pulmonary disease. Although several studies have alluded to the benefits of rehabilitation only a few have been prospective, randomized or controlled. Table I summarizes the five examples of prospective randomized controlled trials of respiratory rehabilitation that we were able to find after conducting a search of the literature published in the last 20 years. When the various protocols are examined in detail their designs limit their generalizability and lead us to conclude that the evidence as to whether respiratory rehabilitation works remains equivocal.

McGavin[1] randomized subjects to an unsupervised exercise program of 3 months duration. Follow-up only occurred when the patients were well, biasing the results since the mean follow-up time for the control group was fourteen weeks compared to nineteen for the exercise group. Sinclair[2] allocated subjects to an exercise or control group according to their residence in or outside of the city. Due to this biased randomization no valid conclusions can be drawn. Cockcroft's[3] study shows the disappearance of a treatment effect over a very short period of time. Improvement in the 12 minute walk was significant at two months, but not at four months because of spontaneous improvements in the untreated controls. Atkins[4] tested a behavioral approach to respiratory rehabilitation incorporating a standardized quality of life instrument into their trial.

The generalizability of their study is questionable since half of the subjects were self-referred, two-thirds were female, and there was a 30% dropout rate by 6

Table I. Controlled studies of respiratory rehabilitation.

	Subjects Treatment	Controls	Randomized	Final outcome	Quality of Life	Cost analysis
McGavin[1]	16	12	Yes	14-19 weeks	Unstandardized	X
3 month unsupervised outpatient program (stairclimbing)						
Sinclair[2]	17	16	No	12 months	Unstandardized	X
Supervised combined in- and outpatient program of variable length (stairclimbing and walking)						
Cockcroft[3]	19	20	Yes	4 months	Unstandardized	X
4 month supervised combined in- and outpatient program (stairclimbing and walking)						
Atkins[4,5]	47	28	Yes	18 months	Standardized	$24,000/
2 month supervised outpatient program (walking and behavior modification)						
Toshima[6]	57	62	Yes	24 months	Standardized	X
2 month supervised outpatient program (education and walking) (controls 8 hours of education)						

months. The first report of an economic analysis of respiratory rehabilitation was undertaken by Toevs[5] using data from the Atkins trial. Toevs estimated that the cost per well year achieved is $24,000 U.S. These costs must be evaluated in the context of the program studied in which five of the six treatment sessions took place in the patient's home.

Toshima[6] has reported preliminary results in an ongoing two year trial with an 89% follow-up rate at six months. In this trial the treatment group was offered an eight week outpatient program (involving 48 hours of education and walking training and weekly group sessions with a psychiatrist), while the control group received 8 hours of education. The preliminary report does not indicate whether an economic evaluation was part of the design.

A common conclusion of these trials is that whereas pulmonary mechanics do not improve, patients do experience an increase in exercise tolerance following a rehabilitation program. How sustainable that increase is remains questionable. Another important conclusion is that patients experience considerable subjective improvement as reflected by a decrease in dyspnea and fatigue and an increase in the ability to perform activities of daily living. Incorporating standardized quality of life measurements in such trials affords a valid and reliable way of assessing these general conclusions.

In addition including a quality of life measurement and/or utility instrument enables investigators to incorporate an economic analysis into a trial.

Having reviewed the literature we became interested in designing a comprehensive trial of respiratory rehabilitation. With the increasing need to justify resource allocation the inclusion of an economic evaluation is highly relevant. The following discussion addresses the principles of economic evaluation, which can be applied to the delivery of any health care treatment.[7, 8]

Economic Evaluation

Those who plan, provide or receive health services face important questions such as:

Should serum cholesterol be checked on every adult?
Should schools run a scoliosis screening program?
Should each piece of new equipment be purchased?
Should public health workers be screened for tuberculosis?

In other words, who should do what to whom and with what health care resources? The answers to these questions are influenced by our estimates of the relative merit of the alternative courses of action. How can the relative merits be established? One type of evaluation is economic.

Before evaluating a Health Service in economic terms one needs to be confident of the answers to the following questions:[9, 10]

1. Can the service work (efficacy) in fully compliant people under optimal circumstances?
2. Does the service work (effectiveness) among those to whom it is offered? Will it be accepted in usual circumstances within the community?
3. Will it reach those who need it (availability)?

Answers to the first two of these questions can be combined in a well designed prospective randomized controlled trial to determine both the relative benefits and costs of respiratory rehabilitation as compared with alternative uses of the same resources.

Why Is Economic Evaluation Important?

Economic analysis is important to clinicians, administrators and policy makers because it affords them an additional tool with which to base decisions on resource allocation.[9, 10] What must be considered in assessing the desirability of a health care program is not just its clinically demonstrated effectiveness but the health outcome achievable in quality adjusted life years (QALY) if the same money were to be used to fund an alternative program (opportunity cost).

Clinicians who commit their time and energy to a particular treatment are usually enthusiastic proponents of that approach. However undertaking an economic evaluation promotes a serious and less biased consideration of the economic merits of various treatment alternatives. For example, if funding for a respiratory rehabilitation program is being considered then valid alternatives (e.g. community care by family physicians) must be given equal consideration.

If the end point is a reduction in morbidity then a logical comparison might well be a smoking cessation program. Thus a clinical trial should take into consideration not only the comprehensive benefit of an isolated program but also the cost of such a program and its alternative.

Lastly, without careful measurement and reporting there may be critical areas of uncertainty regarding costs. A good example of this is the American Cancer Society recommendation that 6 stools be screened for bowel cancer.[11] Everyone recognized that as the number of tests increased, so did the cost. But most people were very surprised to learn that at the time of the sixth test, the cost per case detected was 47 million dollars.

What Is Economic Evaluation?

Definition: *Comparative analysis of alternate courses in terms of costs and benefits.*

The distinguishing characteristics of health care evaluations are that they include both costs and consequences and that they include two or more choices. Therefore the basic steps of any economic evaluation are to identify measure and compare the costs and consequences of the alternatives under consideration.[10] In fact, the characteristics of economic analysis may be used to critique different types of evaluations commonly encountered in the health care literature.

1. Is there a comparison between two or more alternatives?
2. Are both the costs and the consequences considered?

Table II summarizes different types of health care evaluation.[7] The upper part of the table represents only a description because there are no comparisons between existing alternatives. An example of a cost- outcome description might include a coronary care unit in which the results are reported in terms of the costs of operating such a unit and the lives saved.[12]

The unit may be extremely valuable in the treatment of acute myocardial infarction, but in the absence of a comparison with an existing alternative a complete economic evaluation is not possible. In the lower left part of the table (cell 3A), an efficacy evaluation compares two treatments from the point of view of agreed outcome measures but without a cost component. It is this type of evaluation to which most prospective randomized clinical trials belong.

Alternatively one can look just at costs assuming that the outcomes are similar as in a study that compared the costs of providing long term oxygen with cylinders versus a liquid system or concentrators.[13] These types of partial evaluations can be important in assisting clinicians and planners in their understanding of benefits and costs for a particular treatment but they do not attempt to link benefits and costs in measurements that allow for a comprehensive evaluation.

Table II. Distinguishing characteristics of health care evaluation. *Are both costs (inputs) and consequences (outputs) of the alternatives examined?*

	No		Yes
	Examines only consequences	Examines only costs	
No	*1A Partial Evaluation 1B* Outcome Description	Cost Description	*2 Partial Evaluation* Cost-outcome Description
Yes	*3A Partial Evaluation 3B* Efficacy or Effectiveness Evaluation	Cost Analysis	*4 Full Economic Evaluation* Cost-minimization Analysis Cost-effectiveness Analysis Cost-utility Analysis Cost-benefit Analysis

Is there comparison of two or more alternatives

Costs and Consequences in Respiratory Rehabilitation

Costs

Various viewpoints can be adopted when undertaking an economic analysis. In the current instance the question might be "From a societal viewpoint (government or third party funding agencies, patient [direct and indirect costs], specific institution and community) what are the costs and benefits of supervised respiratory rehabilitation in treating patients with COPD compared with the costs and benefits of conventional community care?"

Table III[7] summarizes some of the costs to be considered in the evaluation of a health service. Per diem costing is only an approximate method of measuring what a particular treatment actually costs. Therefore, the first step in undertaking a cost analysis of a treatment is to identify all those who provide direct services to the patient as separate cost centers in order to arrive at a cost per unit of service (for example, the cost per hour of physiotherapy). Secondly, direct costs (wages and supplies) of each service (for example, nursing, physiotherapy, social work) must be determined along with an appropriate basis for allocating capital costs (equipment, buildings, land) and overhead costs (employee benefits, general administration, housekeeping, etc.) to each cost centre. Although complicated and time consuming the resulting data form a solid base from which future economic evaluations or program budgeting can be conducted.

During an ongoing clinical trial it is feasible to gather data from hospital records, medical charts, and patient logs or diaries of the health care services used by patients. Deciding whether or not to include lost productivity costs in an economic evaluation requires careful consideration.[14]

Table III. Costs of health services and programs.

Costs

I. Organizing and operating costs within the health sector
  (e.g. health professionals' time, supplies, equipment, power, capital costs).   *Direct Costs*

II. Costs borne by patients and their families.
  - Out-of-pocket expenses.   - Time lost from work.   *Indirect*
  - Patient and family input into treatment.   - Psychic costs.   *Costs*

III. Costs borne externally to the health sector, patients and their families.

Consequences

Table IV summarizes some of the consequences associated with providing a health service.[7]

Whereas positive changes in laboratory or clinical measurements may be relevant to clinicians, patients are ultimately concerned with decreasing their disability, that is, with functioning at an optimal level. Sophisticated quality of life instruments that are valid, reliable and sensitive have been devised to measure these changes in physical, social and emotional function.

Guyatt[15] and Patrick[16a] have reviewed the types of instruments available to measure quality of life. General health profiles (with well established reliability and validity) allow for a comparison between interventions or conditions. Disease specific instruments are clinically sensitive and more responsive than general health profiles but may be limited in their application for making such comparisons. Utility instruments address the preference of an individual for a particular health status. This preference can be aggregated among a group of individuals to produce a group utility function. Table V lists some of the instruments available. The disease specific instruments listed are the ones designed to be used specifically with the patient population suffering from chronic obstructive pulmonary disease.

Types of Economic Evaluation

There are four main types of economic evaluation.[7] These range from a cost analysis of two treatments without considering benefits, to a comprehensive analysis that allows for the eventual comparison of costs and benefits of treatments among widely differing conditions taking into consideration patient preferences for the benefits achieved. The method of economic analysis chosen should match the questions of interest.

Table IV. Consequences of health services and programs.

Consequences

I. Changes in physical, social and emotional functioning (effects).

II. Changes in resources use (benefits).
     a. For organizing and operating   - For the original condition.
        services within the health sector.   - For unrelated conditions.   *Direct Benefits*

     b. Relating to activities of   - Savings in expenditure or leisure time input.
        patients and their families. - Savings in lost work time   *Indirect Benefits*

III. Changes in the quality of life of patients and families (utility).

Table V. Quality of life instruments.

Health profiles
     - Sickness Impact Profile[18]
     - Functional Limitations Profile (Adaptation of SIP in U.K.)[19]
     - Nottingham Health Profile[20]
     - Quality of Well-Being[21,22]
     - Rand Corporation Instruments[23]

Utility instruments	Specific instruments
- Standard Gamble[24, 25]	- Chronic Respiratory Disease Questionnaire[27, 28]
- Time Trade-Off[26]	- Oxygen Cost Diagram[29]
	- Baseline and Transitional Dyspnea[30]

Cost Minimization Analysis

When two programs have been determined to be similar in outcome, for example, evaluation of overnight gas exchange during sleep, the results may be comparable in every way (namely to generate an accurate polysomnographic record) but one approach requires the establishment of a sleep laboratory and the other an admission to hospital. The focus of this type of cost analysis is on comparison of program costs in monetary terms.

Cost Effectiveness

This approach is applicable if there is a single effect of interest such as prolongation of life. Although this effect may be common to both the alternatives it may be achieved to a different degree. The common unit of measurement could be life-years gained but with differing success and differing costs.

The treatment of choice would not necessarily be the least costly, but rather the treatment that provides the best cost per effect. For example, it might be the cost per disability day saved when one compares long term inhaled high dose steroids with conventional bronchodilator treatment for asthma. Before making such comparisons it is very important to determine that similar measurement approaches are applied to both limbs of the study.

Cost Benefit Analysis

If the benefits of treatment are evaluated using different units a common denominator is lacking. For example, life-years gained as a result of a smoking cessation program versus disability days saved as a result of influenza-immunization. Under these circumstances the benefits may be translated into monetary terms. A cost benefit analysis although acceptable to an economist may be very much less attractive to health care workers because of the difficulty in translating clinical benefits into purely monetary units.

Cost Utility

Cost utility analysis is based on the economic concept of utility value that reflects the level of satisfaction experienced by a consumer.[16b] In the health care setting utilities are "the numbers that represent the strength of the individual's preference for particular outcomes when faced with uncertainty".[17]

Cost effectiveness analysis can be converted to cost utility analysis with the incorporation of utility instruments allowing life-years gained to be reported as quality adjusted life-years (QALY).

Table V lists the two utility instruments most commonly used. The difference between a measurement of quality of life and the utility of that measurement is contingent on the significance that different individuals may place on the same health status. If for example, identical twins - one a historian and the other a sprinter - were to have pneumonectomies, although clinically their post operative health status may be equivalent, the utility of the treatment may be quite different for the one able to continue work as a historian than for the sprinter who would have to abandon racing.

Conclusion

It is likely that respiratory rehabilitation programs are useful in the long term management of patients with chronic obstructive pulmonary disease. Despite the large volume of anecdotal reports only a few studies have been prospective randomized and controlled. Only one or two have added standardized quality of life measurements to the usual laboratory measurements of physiology and exercise. None have incorporated utility measurements.

Only in a controlled randomized trial that incorporates both the costs and benefits of two or more treatments can the comprehensive merits of those treatments be determined. Economic analysis should be seen as a tool to augment rather than replace current approaches to priorizing health care which will still include ethical considerations, philosophies of social responsibility, political issues and common sense.

Acknowledgement

This work is supported by the West Park Hospital Foundation, the Ontario Ministry of Health Rehabilitation Development and Technology Consortium and the Respiratory Health Network of Centres of Excellence.

References

1. McGavin C., Gupta S.P., Lloyd E.L., McHardy G.J.: Physical Rehabilitation for the Chronic Bronchitic: Results of a Controlled Trial of Exercises in the Home. Thorax, 1977; 32:307-311
2. Sinclair D.J.M., Ingram C.G.: Controlled Trial of Supervised Exercise Training in Chronic Bronchitis. Br. Med. J. 1980; 23:519-521
3. Cockcroft A.E., Saunders M.J., Berry G.: Randomized Controlled Trial of Rehabilitation in Chronic Respiratory Disability. Thorax 1981; 36:200-203
4. Atkins C.J., Kaplan R.M., Timms R.M., Reinsch S., Lofback D.: Behavioral Exercise Programs in theManagement of Chronic Obstructive Pulmonary Disease. J. Consult. Clin. Psychol. 1984; 52, 4:591-603
5. Toevs C.D., Kaplan R.M., Atkins C.J.: The Costs and Effects of Behavioral Programs in Chronic Obstructive Pulmonary Disease. Med. Care 1984; 22, 12:1088-1100
6. Toshima M.T., Kaplan, R.M., Ries, A.: Experimental Evaluation of Rehabilitation in Chronic Obstructive Pulmonary Disease: Short-Term Effects on Exercise Endurance and Health Status. Health Psychol. 1990; 9, 3:237-252
7. Drummond M.F., Stoddart G.L., Torrance G.W.: *Methods for the Economic Evaluation of Health Care Programs.* Oxford: Oxford University Press, 1986
8. Boyle M.H., Torrance G.W., Horwood S.P., Sinclair J.C.: A Cost Analysis for Providing Neonatal Intensive Care to 500-1499 Gram Birth Weight Infants - Research Report #51, Program for Quantitative Studies in Economics and Population. Hamilton, McMaster University, Ontario, Canada, 1982
9. Detsky A.S., Naglie I.G.: A Clinician's Guide to Cost Effectiveness Analysis. Ann. Intern. Med. 1990; 113: 147-154
10. Department of Clinical Epidemiology and Biostatistics. How to Read Clinical Journals VII. To Understand and economic evaluation (Part A). Can. Med. Ass. J., 1984; 130: 1428-1433. (Part B) 1542-1549
11. Neuhauser D., Lewicki A M.: What Do We Gain from a 6th Stool Guaiac. New Eng. J. Med., 1975; 293: 226-228
12. Reynell P.C., Reynell M.C.: The Cost Benefit Analysis of a Coronary Care Unit. Br. Heart J., 1972; 34:897-900

46

13. Lowson K.V., Drummond M.F., Bishop J.M.: Costing New Services: Long Term Domiciliary Oxygen Therapy. Lancet, 1981; 2:1146-1149

14. Grabowski H.G., Hansen R.W.: Economic Scales and Tests. In: B. Spilker (Ed.) *Quality of Life Assessments in Clinical Trials*. New York, Raven Press, 1990

15. Guyatt G.M., Valdhuyzen Van Zanten S.J.O., Feeny D.H., Patrick D.L: Measuring Quality of Life in Clinical Trials: A Taxonomy and Review. Can. Med. Ass. J., 1989; 40:1441-1448

16. Patrick D.L, Deyo R.A.: Generic and Disease Specific Measures in Assessing. Health Status and Quality of Life. Medical Care, 1989; 27, 3: S217-S232

16. Feeny D.H., Labelle R., Torrance G.W.: Integrating Economic Evaluations and Quality of Life Assessments. In: B. Spilker (Ed.) *Quality of Life Assessments in Clinical Trials*. New York, Raven Press, 1990

17. Torrance G.W., Feeny D.: Utilities and Quality-Adjusted Life Years. Intern. J. Technol. Assess. Health Care, 1989; 5: 559-575

18. Bergner M., Bobbitt R.A, Carter W.B., Gilson B.S.: The Sickness Impact Profile Development and Final Revision of a Health Status Measure. Medical Care, 1981; 19, 8: 787-805

19. Patrick D.L, Sittampalam Y., Somerville S.M., Carter W.B., Bergner M. A: Cross-Cultural Comparison of Health Status Values. Am. J. Public Health, 1985; 75, 12: 1402-1407

20. Hunt S., McEwen J., McKenna S.P.: Nottingham Health Profile. In: S. Hunt, J. McEwen, S.P. McKenna (Eds.) *Measuring Health Status*. London, Croom Helm 1986

21. Kaplan R.M., Atkins C.J., Timms R.: Validity of a Quality of Well-Being Scale as an Outcome Measure in Chronic Obstructive Pulmonary Disease. J. Chronic Dis., 1984; 37, 2: 85-95

22. Kaplan R.M., Anderson J.P.: The Quality of Well Being Scale: Rationale for a Single Quality of Life Index. In: S.R. Walker, R.M. Rosser (Eds.) *Quality of Life: Assessment and Application*. Lancaster, MTP Press, 1988

23. Ware J.E., et al.: *Conceptualization and Measurement of Physiological Health for Adults in the Health Insurance Study. Vol. 1. Model of Health and Methodology*. Santa Monica CA, Rand Corporation, 1980

24. Torrance G.W.: Measurement of Health State Utilities for Economic Appraisal. J. Health Econ., 1986; 5: 1-30

25. Capwell G.: Techniques of Health Status Measurement Using a Health Index. In: G. Teeling Smith (Ed.) *Measuring Health: A Practical Approach*. Chichester, John Wiley, 1988

26. Buxton M., Ashby J.: The Time-Trade-Off Approach to Health State Evaluation. In: G. Teeling Smith (Ed.) *Measuring Health: A Practical Approach*. Chichester, John Wiley, 1988

27. Guyatt G.: Measuring Health Status in Chronic Airflow Limitation. Eur. Resp. J., 1988; 1: 560-564

28. Guyatt G., et al.: A New Measure of Quality of Life for Clinical Trials in Chronic Lung Disease. Thorax, 1987; 42 (10): 773-778

29. McGavin C.R., Artvinli M., Naoe H., McHardy G.J.R.: Dyspnea, Disability and Distamce Walked: Comparison of Estimates of Exercise Performance in Respiratory Disease. B.M.J., 1978; 22: 241-243

30. Mahler D.A., Weinberg D.H., Wells C.K., Feinstein A.R. The Measurement of Dyspnea: Contents. Interobserver Agreement, and Physiologic Correlates of Two New Clinical Indexes. Chest, 1984; 85, 6: 751-758

Evaluation

5. Respiratory Function Tests in Pulmonary Rehabilitation

C. RAMPULLA, N. AMBROSINO, C. FRACCHIA, R. CORSICO

Fondazione Clinica del Lavoro, IRCCS, Centro Medico di Riabilitazione di Montescano, Pavia, Italy

Respiratory rehabilitation programs are widely employed in the management of patients with respiratory diseases. Nevertheless only few prospective, randomized or controlled studies have been performed on these programs and their clinical efficacy is still debated. A survey of literature in this field shows that many studies evaluated the effects of some of these programs performing respiratory function tests measuring parameters which the specific maneuvers studied were not objectively able to influence. In other words each maneuver of chest physiotherapy should be evaluated with specific tests.

Pulmonary rehabilitation for patients with chronic lung diseases included interventions designed to improve bronchial clearance, to optimize the position of the diaphragm, breathing exercise, physical exercise and respiratory muscle training and more recently non-invasive mechanical ventilation.[1-3]

Chest Physiotherapy

Chest physiotherapy includes all techniques aimed at removing secretions from the airways. The most widely used technique is postdural drainage. Refinement of chest physiotherapy has led to the development of the active cycle of breathing exercises including the forced expiration technique.[4,5]

The objectives of this classical technique are to enhance mucociliary clearance to reduce airway obstruction and increase airflows. The effects of this technique have been assessed in terms of amount of daily sputum. As a rule bronchial drainage is performed when patients show a spontaneous daily sputum production greater than 30 ml. The value of this measurement is questionable; in fact many practical problems (ability to collect sputum, amount of ingested sputum etc.) make this measurement rather insensitive. On the other hand, measurement of rheologic properties of sputum are difficult, time consuming and expensive.

Measurements of airflow by means of FVC and FEV_1 has been shown to change little following postural drainage, and in some cases these parameters worsen so that inhalation of bronchodilators is advised before submission to these maneuvers. Monitoring of oxygen saturation and heart should be performed during the execution of chest physiotherapy sessions.

Blood gas analysis has proven to be not very useful in the assessment of the efficacy of bronchial drainage. Increasing airway clearance should effect a better distribution of ventilation. This does not automatically imply an improvement in blood gases. In fact if better distribution of ventilation does not match with an improvement in perfusion of the same lung zones, this would result in a worsening of blood gases.

Breathing Exercises

The objectives of this technique are mainly to put the diaphragm in a better situation of its length-tension relationship in order to increase its efficiency. Minute ventilation, blood gas analysis, movement of the diaphragm as assessed by roentgenoscopy have been used to evaluate the efficacy of this technique, but the most specific measurement should be diaphragmatic strength, and subjective evaluation of dyspnea. The main goal of these exercises is to teach a low frequency high tidal volume pattern of breathing, especially in patients with COPD. Tidal volume, minute ventilation and blood gas analysis have been performed to evaluate the effects, but often results do not fit with the subjective benefits of these techniques in term of dyspnea and ability to cope with day to day activities. Exercise tolerance does not seem to be a sensitive index to assess the effects of these exercises, while no change in spirometry has been reported.[6,7]

Both these two techniques work by changing the breathing pattern of the patients. Monitoring of breathing pattern is the best way to evaluate the effects of these techniques. It is well known that a mouthpiece can affect breathing pattern per se. Non-invasive methods of evaluation of breathing pattern have been shown to be sensitive enough to avoid use of a mouthpiece, or to measure ventilation in conditions such as effort, disease or sleep.

Respiratory inductive plethysmography and magnetometry have been used for this purpose. At the moment their use is limited to study purposes, but they may be used as a tool for biofeedback techniques with the aim of teaching patients a new breathing pattern. Both respiratory inductive plethysmography and magnetometry assess non-invasively (without mouthpiece) ventilation by measuring rib cage and abdomen motion during each breathing act. Non-invasive assessment of ventilation has been performed during a session of breathing training. Analysis of rib cage and abdomen during inspiration which has been attributed to inspiratory muscle fatigue. By means of these methods, rapid shallow breathing can be recorded and the effects of therapy, if any, can be documented.[8]

Whole Body and Skeletal Muscle Exercises

Severe chronic airflow limitation is associated with chronic disability and handicap. Functional exercise capacity and gases exchange but as these induce a reduction in daily activities muscle function is also reduced, which may eventually become a limiting factor. General muscle fatigue has been considered as the limiting symptom of maximal exercise capacity in almost a third of COPD patients. Measurements of isometric strength of quadriceps muscle, handgrip and respiratory muscle indicate that reduction in ventilatory capacity is accompanied by reduction in skeletal muscle strength which may contribute indipendently to reductions in exercise capacity.

Exercise rehabilitation programs have been performed in the hope that improvements in exercise capacity might be achieved, despite the absence of any expected effect on pulmonary function, but the results have been variable with only modest improvements in aerobic capacity being found.[9-12]

Neither respiratory muscle function nor lung function tests have been reported to be influenced by exercise training. Quality of life indexes should be better indicators of usefulness of this technique. Weightlifting exercise training has been shown to be effective in patients with chronic airflow limitation, with benefits in muscle strength, exercise endurance and subjective responses to some of the demands of daily living.[13-14]

Respiratory Muscle Training

Both strength and endurance of respiratory muscle have been shown to improve in response to specific training programs.[15] It has been suggested that strengthening the respiratory muscle in patients with chronic airflow limitation may reduce the discomfort of daily activities and increase functional capacity. Some studies have reported improved respiratory muscle strength and endurance, improved exercise capacity and improved functional capacity and reduced dyspnea in day to day life following respiratory muscle training.

These studies have been limited by inadequate controls, lack of placebo and small sample size. Some authors report increases in exercise tolerance but probably the most useful indexes of efficacy should be quality of life, capacity for activities of daily living as assessed by walking distance test, and assessment of dyspnea. Reduction in $PaCO_2$ might be a goal of inspiratory muscle strength.

Respiratory muscle strength is usually evaluated by assessment of maximal static inspiratory and expiratory pressures, while maximal voluntary ventilation, maximal sustained ventilatory capacity, time of maintenance of breathing at a given fraction of maximal inspiratory pressure, and the highest resistive or threshold load that can be sustained for 10 minutes have been used to assess inspiratory muscle endurance training.[16,17]

Respiratory Muscle Rest Techniques

Inspiratory muscle fatigue may be a cause of hypercapnic respiratory failure. Muscle fatigue is defined as a condition in which there is a loss in the capacity for developing force and/or velocity in response to a load and which is reversible by rest.[18]

Mechanical ventilation in non-invasive ways is being increasingly employed in the treatment of chronic hypercapnic respiratory insufficiency with the aim of improving arterial blood gases and "resting" inspiratory muscles.[16]

Pulmonary function, especially VC, FEV_1, MVV, blood gas analysis and assessment of respiratory muscle function should be evaluated to include patients in programs of treatment with mechanical ventilation. Pulmonary function test, blood gases, respiratory muscle strength and endurance, cardiac output, sleep studies and electromyographic evaluation of respiratory muscle should be assessed before starting treatment.

The effectiveness of such techniques should be assessed obviously by determination of blood gas analysis both during ventilation and at long term. Effective inspiratory muscle rest should be assessed by evaluating the reduction of integrated surface electromyographic activity. Improvement in inspiratory muscle strength and ability to cope with daily activities as assessed by quality of life questionnaires and walking test, should also be monitored especially in case of long term domiciliary mechanical ventilation.

Symptomatic demonstration of the usefulness of the treatment may be necessary to encourage patients use mechanical ventilation.[19,20]

References

1. Rochester D.F., Goldberg S.K.: Techniques of respiratory physical therapy. Am. Rev. Respir. Dis. 1980; 122(5), Part 2: 133-146
2. Donner C.F., Howard P.: Pulmonary rehabilitation in chronic obstructive pulmonary disease (COPD) with recommendations for its use. Eur. Respir. J. 1992; 5: 266-275
3. American Thoracic Society: Standards for the diagnosis and care of patients with chronic obstructive pulmonary disease and asthma. Am. Rev. Respir. Dis. 1987; 136: 255-274
4. Webber B.A., Hodson M.E., Batten J.C.: Evaluation of the forced expiration technique as an adjunct to postural drainage in the treatment of cystic fibrosis. Br. Med. J. 1979; 2: 417-418

5. Selsby D.S.: Chest physiotherapy. Br. Med. J. 1989; 298: 541-542

6. Sergysels R., Willeput R., Lenders D., Vachaudez J.P., Schandevyl W., Hennebert A.: Low frequency breathing at rest and during exercise in severe chronic obstructive bronchitis. Thorax, 1979; 34: 536-539

7. Erpicum B., Willeput R., Sergysels R.: Does abdominal breathing below FRC give a mechanical support for inspiration? Clin. Respir. Physiol. 1984; 20: 117

8. Konno K., Mead J.: Measurements of separate volume changes of rib cage and abdomen during breathing. J. Appl. Physiol. 1967; 22: 407-422

9. Keens T.G., Krastins I.R.B., Wannamaker E.M., Levison H., Crozier D.N., Bryan A.C.: Ventilatory muscle endurance training in normal subjects and patients with cystic ficbrosis. Am. Rev. Respir. Dis. 1977; 116: 853-860

10. Belman H.J., Kendregan B.A.: Physical training fails to improve ventilatory muscle endurance in patients with chronic obstructive pulmonary disease. Chest 1982; 81: 440-443

11. Celli B., Criner G., Rassulo J.: Ventilatory muscle recruitment during unsupported arm exercise in normal subjects. J. Appl. Physiol. 1988; 64: 1936-1941

12. Simpson K., Killian K., McCartney N., Stubbing D.G., Jones N.L.: Randomized controlled trial of weightlifting exercise in patients with chronic airflow limitation. Thorax, 1992; 47: 70-75

13. McGavin C.R., Gupta S.P., McHardy G.J.: Twelve-minute walking test for assessing disability in chronic bronchitis. Br. Med. J. 1978; i: 822-823

14. Guyatt G., Berman L.B., Townsend M., Pugsley S.O., Chambers L.W.: A measure of quality of life for clinical trials in chronic lung disease. Thorax, 1987; 42: 773-778

15. Leith D.E., Bradley M.E.: Ventilatory muscle strength and endurance training. J. Appl. Physiol. 1976; 41: 508-516

16. Rampulla C., Ambrosino N.: Inspiratory muscle training and rest in COPD patients. Eur. Respir. Rev. 1991; 1: 490-497

17. Smith K., Cook D.J., Guyatt G.H., Madhaven J., Oxman A.D.: Respiratory muscle training in chronic airflow limitation: a metanalysis. Am. Rev. Respir. Dis. 1992; 145: 533-539

18. NHLBI workshop summary. Respiratory muscle fatigue. Report of the Respiratory Muscle Fatigue Workshop Group. Am. Rev. Respir. Dis. 1990; 142: 474-480

19. Fracchia C., Ambrosino N.: Negative-pressure ventilation. RT International 1992; (August): 39-42

20. Nava S., Ambrosino N., Zocchi L., Rampulla C.: Diaphragmatic rest during negative pressure ventilation by pneumowrap. Assessment in normal and COPD patients. Chest 1990; 98: 857-865

6. Dyspnea Scores

J.W. FITTING

Division of Pneumology, Department of Internal Medicine, Chuv, Lausanne, Switzerland

Introduction

Dyspnea is a prominent complaint and a frequent cause of exercise limitation in patients with chronic respiratory diseases. It is therefore desirable to estimate this symptom quantitatively in order to better assess the functional impairment and the effects of treatment in these patients. Because dyspnea, or breathlessness, corresponds to a sensation, its measurement cannot be as straightforward as those of objective variables. However, certain instruments have been developed to this end which enable us to quantify dyspnea and to relate it to other respiratory parameters.

Definition of Dyspnea

Before attempting to measure dyspnea, one should agree on what is to be measured. Indeed, the term dyspnea may convey slightly different meanings. In the literature dyspnea has been variably defined as "a feeling of an uncomfortable need to breathe", "a sensation of experiencing air hunger", "a sensation of labored or difficult breathing", "an unpleasant awareness of breathing and of respiratory distress", or "an uncomfortable awareness of breathing or an increased respiratory effort that is unpleasant and regarded as inappropriate".

Simon et al.[1] recently addressed the question of whether dyspnea might encompass different types of sensations. In normal subjects submitted to eight different respiratory stimuli, different qualities of sensations were evoked. Among the most physiologic stimuli, elastic loading elicited a sensation of air hunger, resistive loading elicited sensations of air hunger and increased respiratory effort, whereas exercise elicited sensations of rapid and heavy breathing.[1] The possible qualitative variability of dyspnea should be taken into account when measurements are undertaken, particularly in prospective studies. One option is to precisely define the sensation that is to be rated by the subject. Another option is to ask for scoring dyspnea or breathlessness without further definition. These experimental conditions should be consistent throughout the study and should be explicitly reported.

Indirect Measurement of Dyspnea

The assessment of dyspnea can be attempted by indirect or by direct measurements. The indirect measurements are based on questionnaires assessing the exercise tolerance and functional impairment of the subject. These indirect scores quantify the level of exercise that is limited by dyspnea but do not provide quantification of dyspnea itself.

Direct Measurement of Dyspnea: Ratio Scales

The direct measurement of dyspnea relies on the techniques of psychophysics, which is the quantitative study of the relationship between sensory stimuli and the evoked sensory response. Among different related techniques, the open magnitude scales have been widely used. They represent ratio scales of apparent magnitude where the subject estimates the intensity of his subjective impressions by freely attributing numbers. Having experienced an initial stimulus, the subject must rate a series of stimuli of different intensities by choosing numbers in proportion to his subjective impressions. These scales are termed open because the subjects are not limited in their ratings. The utilization of these scales showed that all sensory modes obey a power function, as described by Stevens.[2,3]

The perceived magnitude (Ψ) of a stimulus is related to the intensity (Φ) of the stimulus by the following equation: $\Psi = k\Phi^n$ (Stevens's law).

The exponent (n) thus describes the shape of the psychophysical relationship of a given sensory mode, or its dynamic operating characteristics. When the exponent is < 1 the sensation grows as a decelerating function with respect to the physical stimulus, as for the sense of light brightness (n = 0.33).

When n = 1 the sensation grows as a linear function, as for the visual estimation of length. When n is >1 the sensation grows as an accelerating function, as for electric shocks (n = 3.5).[2,3] The sense of effort during exertion also grows as an accelerating function with n = 1.6.[4]

In the pursuit of the underlying mechanisms of dyspnea, open magnitude scaling has been used to characterize the sensory response to respiratory loads. Killian et al. [5] thus demonstrated that the perceived magnitude (Ψ) of added loads is not dependent on the load itself, resistive or elastic, but rather on the inspiratory pressure (P) and its duration (t): $\Psi = k\, p^{1.3}\, t^{0.56}$. This technique has also been used to determine whether patients with chronic lung diseases manifest an impaired perception of added loads in comparison with age-matched normal subjects. The results were however contradictory.[6, 7]

The main limitation of ratio scales is their inability to compare individual responses in absolute values. If the shape of the relationship between dyspnea and loads or exertion can be established, the assessment of the absolute degree of dyspnea is impossible. The interval scales were developed in order to obviate this limitation.

Direct Measurement of Dyspnea: Interval Scales

With interval scales, the subject is asked to partition a closed scale into equal-appearing intervals. Two widely used scales belong to this category: the Visual Analog Scale (VAS) and the Borg scale.

a. Visual Analog Scale

The Visual Analog Scale (VAS) consists of a 10 or 20 cm straight line whose extremities are marked by the two descriptors "not at all breathless" and "extremely breathless" (Fig. 1). The subject rates his dyspnea by simply indicating a point on the line. Dyspnea may conveniently be measured at intervals of one minute during an exercise test. The handling of the VAS is affected by the individual perception of the minimum and maximum points. If "not at all breathless" can be related to the resting state, the notion "extremely breathless" is likely to depend on several factors including the usual level of physical activity.

Different methods may be used to "calibrate" the maximum point. A prior strenuous exercise may be accomplished in order to anchor the perception of extreme breathlessness. It is important that dyspnea be greater during this procedure than during the test itself. However, the sensitivity of the VAS will be reduced if dyspnea during this prior exercise greatly exceeds that expected during the main test.[8] It is not necessary to repeat this calibration test before each study as the perception of maximum breathlessness remains stable over one month.[9] In practice, however, it is often difficult to impose such a strenuous prior exercise to dyspneic patients. Another way to anchor the perception of maximum consists in relating it to an activity performed by the patient in his daily life and which is associated with an easily recalled severe breathlessness.[10]

The reproducibility of the VAS has been tested after various intervals. The VAS score was recorded minute by minute during progressive treadmill exercise in healthy subjects. No significant difference was found at any point when the test was repeated after one week.[8] The reproducibility of the VAS was assessed in normal subjects submitted either to progressive or to intermittent hypercapnia. The VAS

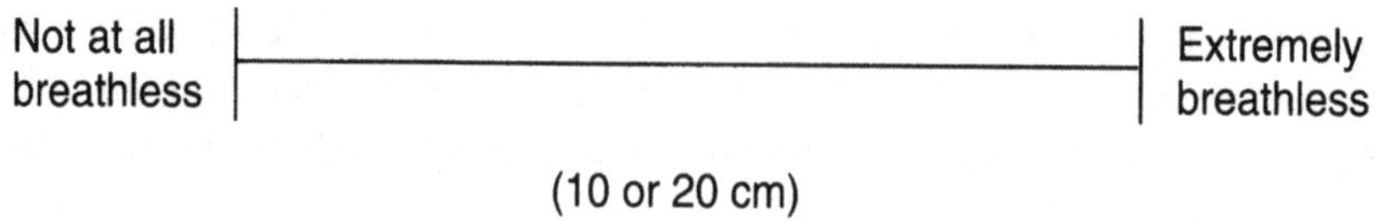

Not at all breathless		Extremely breathless

(10 or 20 cm)

Fig. 1. Visual Analog Scale (VAS).

scores were compared at matched levels of minute ventilation. During progressive hypercapnia, reproducibility was good after one day and one week, but poor after one year, as judged by correlation coefficients.

During intermittent ventilatory stimulation the reproducibility was also good after one day and one week.[11] In patients with COPD exercising on a treadmill, the reproducibility of VAS scores was deemed adequate after five days, as based on a qualitative analysis.[10]

Another study assessed the reproducibility of VAS scores during progressive cycling exercise in patients with various chronic lung diseases, on three occasions within two weeks. In 12 out of 13 patients, the mean standard deviation of repeated individual VAS scores at isopower output was 8%.[9] In these studies a minority of patients showed poorly reproducible results. It follows that the individual reproducibility of VAS scores should be determined before including patients in a prospective study.[12]

One important limitation of the VAS lies in the individual variability in the use of the scale. Indeed, healthy subjects and patients may use the full range of the scale, or only part of it, in a personal way.[8, 10-13] Thus, the VAS allows intrasubject comparisons of dyspnea between different conditions, but it does not permit comparisons between individuals.

Another theoretical drawback of the VAS lies in its distortion of the actual psychophysical relationship.

When compared with open magnitude scales, interval scales always yield a lower increase in perceived magnitude for a given increase in physical magnitude. In other words, the interval scales are characterized by a lower exponent (n), which has been termed the virtual exponent in opposition with the actual exponent obtained with open magnitude scaling.[14, 15]

b. Borg Scale

Borg designed a scale to obviate the kind of limitations shared by the VAS.[16] The Borg scale (sometimes called the modified Borg scale with reference to a previous version) is composed of numbers from 0 to 10 (Fig. 2). A series of descriptive terms is attached to numbers.

These terms, "slight", "moderate", "severe", etc. have been chosen according to their general use in different sensory modes. Their purpose is to improve the understanding of the scale and to favor a more uniform handling of the scale by different individuals. As it happens, most subjects are able to understand and to handle the scale easily. Furthermore, the Borg scale was designed to restore the actual psychophysical relationship and the accelerating function of dyspnea. For instance, "moderate" is not attached to 5 at mid-scale, but to 3. Thus, the Borg scale represents an interval scale with some ratio properties.

The reproducibility of the Borg scale was assessed in COPD patients exercising on a bicycle ergometer. During tests repeated after one hour, and one to ten days, there was no significant difference in Borg score either at two minutes or at maximal exercise. Moreover, the mean intrasubject coefficient of variation of Borg score was not significantly different from those of maximal minute ventilation and maximal oxygen consumption.[17]

The VAS and the Borg scale were compared in normal subjects exercising repeatedly with increasing and decreasing workloads on a bicycle ergometer. In general, the individual subjects used the two scales in a similar manner but showed some interindividual differences.

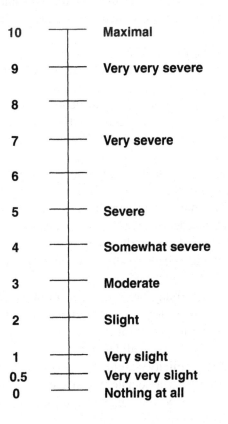

Fig. 2. Borg scale.

Both scales showed a correlation between dyspnea and minute ventilation, which however was tighter with the Borg scale.

Dyspnea was lower on a second test performed 2-6 weeks later, but the difference was less marked with the Borg scale than with the VAS. Thus, the two scales appeared valid, with some advantage for the Borg scale which showed slightly better reproducibility and closer correlation with minute ventilation.[18]

Application of Dyspnea Scores

Several psychophysical techniques are available for the measurement of dyspnea, each of them being characterized by its own strengths and limitations. The selection of a scale depends on the question that is being addressed.

If the study aims at determining the true shape of the relationship between a stimulus and dyspnea, then open magnitude scaling must be used. If dyspnea is to be assessed in absolute value and compared across different conditions or individuals the VAS or the Borg scale are far more practical, if not entirely valid.

The VAS and the Borg scale are useful to measure dyspnea on exertion, either in case of dyspnea of unknown origin or in the assessment of functional impairment of patients with known respiratory disorders.

Dyspnea is usually scored at one minute intervals during an incremental exercise test. The VAS or Borg scores can then be plotted versus power output or oxygen consumption.[9,17,19]

Because dyspnea is closely linked to minute ventilation ($\dot{V}E$) in normal subjects and in respiratory patients,[8,10-12,17,18] the diagram dyspnea-$\dot{V}E$ is of interest. First, it can be used in pharmacological studies to distinguish different drug effects on breathlessness.

A drug can potentially decrease dyspnea in two ways: either by decreasing $\dot{V}E$, or by decreasing the slope of the dyspnea-$\dot{V}E$ relationship.[12] Second, a diminution of the dyspnea-$\dot{V}E$ slope may also reflect changes in mechanical properties of the respiratory system, such as a decrease in lung resistance and elastance or an increase in respiratory muscle strength and endurance.

The Borg scores have also been related to other respiratory parameters in an attempt to explore the mechanisms of dyspnea.

Thus, during loaded breathing the sense of respiratory effort correlated with mouth pressure,[20] pleural pressure,[21, 22] and sternocleidomastoid EMG activity,[23] but not with the diaphragmatic tension-time index[21] or EMG activity.[23] In summary, instruments exist and have been validated for the measurement of dyspnea. However, their apparent simplicity should not lead to overlooking the limitations and methodological questions associated with each of these scales. Reliable measurements of dyspnea can be obtained with minimal hardware but they require some knowledge of psychophysical rules.

References

1. Simon P.M., Schwarzstein R.M., Weiss J.W., Lahive K., Fencl V., Teghtsoonian M., Weinberger S.E.: Distinguishable sensations of breathlessness induced in normal volunteers. Am. Rev. Respir. Dis. 1988; 140:1021-1027

2. Stevens S.S.: On the psychophysical law. Psychol. Rev. 1957; 64:153-181

3. Stevens S.S.: *Psychophysics*. Ed. by G. Stevens. Chichester, John Wiley and Sons, 1975

4. Borg GAV, Noble BJ: Perceived exertion. Exercise and Sports Science Reviews 1974; 2:131-153

5. Killian KJ, Bucens DD, Campbell EJM: Effect of breathing patterns on the perceived magnitude of added loads to breathing. J. Appl. Physiol. 1982; 52:578-584

6. Ward ME, Stubbing DG: Effect of chronic lung disease on the perception of added inspiratory loads. Am. Rev. Respir. Dis. 1985; 132:652-656

7. Gottfried SB, Redline S, Altose MD: Respiratory sensation in chronic obstructive pulmonary disease. Am. Rev. Respir. Dis. 1985; 132:954-959

8. Stark RD, Gambles SA, Lewis JA: Methods to assess breathlessness in healthy subjects: a critical evaluation and application to analyse the acute effects of diazepam and promethazine on breathlessness induced by exercise or by exposure to raised levels of carbon dioxide. Clin. Sci. 1981; 61:429-439

9. Loiseau A, Dubreuil C, Pujet JC: Echelle visuelle analogique de dyspnée a l'exercise. Rev. Mal. Resp. 1990; 7:39-44

10. Stark RD, Gambles SA, Chatterjee SS: An exercise test to assess clinical dyspnoea: estimation of reproducibility and sensitivity. Br. J. Dis. Chest 1982; 76:269-278

11. Adams L, Chronos N, Lane R, Guz A: The measurement of breathlessness induced in normal subjects: validity of two scaling techniques. Clin. Sci. 1985; 69:7-16

12. Stark RD: Dyspnoea: assessment and pharmacological manipulation. Eur. Respir. J. 1988; 1:280-287

13. Adams L, Chronos N, Lane R, Guz A:The measurement of breathlessness induced in normal subjects: individual differences. Clin. Sci. 1986; 70:131-140

14. Stevens SS: Issues in psychophysical measurement. Psychol. Rev. 1971; 78:426-450

15. Killian KJ: Assessment of dyspnoea. Eur. Respir. J. 1988; 1:195-197

16. Borg GAV: Psychophysical bases of perceived exertion. Med. Sci. Sports Exercise 1982; 14:377-381

17. Silverman M, Barry J, Hellerstein H, Janos J, Kelsen S: Variability of the perceived sense of effort in breathing during exercise in patients with chronic obstructive pulmonary disease. Am. Rev. Respir. Dis. 1988; 137:206-209

18. Wilson RC, Jones PW: A comparison of the visual analogue scale and modified Borg scale for the measurement of dyspnoea during exercise. Clin. Sci. 1989; 76:277-282

19. Leblanc P, Bowie DM, Summers E, Jones NL, Killian KJ: Breathlessness and exercise in patients with cardiorespiratory disease. Am. Rev. Respir. Dis. 1986; 133:21-25

20. Jones GL, Killian KJ, Summers E, Jones NL: Inspiratory muscle forces and endurance in maximum resistive loading. J. Appl. Physiol. 1985; 58:1608-1615

21. Bradley TD, Chartrand DA, Fitting JW, Killian KJ, Grassino A: The relation of inspiratory effort sensation to fatiguing patterns of the diaphragm. Am. Rev. Respir. Dis. 1986; 134:1119-1124

22. Fitting JW, Chartrand DA, Bradley TD, Killian KJ, Grassino A: Effect of thoracoabdominal breathing patterns on inspiratory effort sensation. J. Appl. Physiol. 1987; 62:1665-1670

23. Ward ME, Eidelman D, Stubbing DG, Bellemare F, Macklem PT: Respiratory sensation and pattern of respiratory muscle activation during diaphragm fatigue. J. Appl. Physiol. 1988; 65: 2181-2189

7. Exercise Limitation in Pulmonary Rehabilitation

A.G. Stewart, P. Howard

Department of Medicine and Pharmacology, University of Sheffield, Royal Hallamshire Hospital, Sheffield, United Kingdom

Therapy for the relief of dyspnea in patients with chronic obstructive pulmonary disease (COPD) is primarily aimed at reducing reversible airflow obstruction with bronchodilator drugs, preventing or promptly treating infections and correcting hypoxemia through the use of oxygen where appropriate. Exercise training has the potential to improve exercise endurance and reduce exertional dyspnea.[1]

The level of work required for training varies. Most workers agree that work rate needs to be above that of the anaerobic (lactate) threshold (AT). Casaburi et al.[1] showed that COPD patients using a training program above their pre training AT raised the level of the AT with a consequent reduction in lactate production and a reduced ventilatory requirement.

These patients were able to maintain physical work at levels above their pretraining anaerobic threshold. In comparison an age, sex and severity of disease matched group of COPD controls who performed the same amount of work but at a lower work rate such that they did not reach their anaerobic threshold showed little improvement in ventilation, lactate production or endurance when exercised above their pretraining anaerobic threshold at the end of the rehabilitation program. In normal persons and patients a physiological training effect only occurs when the work rate exceeds that at the anaerobic threshold. Work rates below the anaerobic threshold may sustain rather than improve fitness.[2-4] Although physiological limits in COPD patients may not be improved, there are still benefits. Regular exercise improves the quality of life by the patient learning more skilful ways of performing physical tasks, patients may lose weight and thereby increase maximum work output and finally, the psychological improvements gained from regular exercise are well recognized.

Unfortunately, many patients are unable to reach the anaerobic threshold due to the severity of their disease. Furthermore, the absolute level of anaerobic threshold is very variable in patients with COPD and may vary with degree of hypoxemia and also during episodes of pulmonary decompensation.

Patients with respiratory disease have a number of pathologies limiting exercise (Tab. I). These will be discussed.

Table I Limitations to exercise.

1. Ventilatory	3. $\dot{V}/\dot{Q}$ inequality	5. Psychological
2. Circulatory	4. Muscular	

Ventilatory Limitation

The major component of exercise limitation in respiratory disease is reduced ventilatory capacity[5] (Table II) through obstructive or restrictive defects. Dyspnea is associated with an inability to increase ventilation during exercise and to clear excess carbon dioxide.[6,7] In COPD marked reduction in maximum expiratory flow rate at all lung volumes is seen. In emphysema, this is due to increased airway obstruction coupled with reduced elastic recoil. In asthma and chronic bronchitis airways resistance is elevated and hyperinflation means that inspiratory muscles work at a mechanical disadvantage. Expiratory times are prolonged, encroaching on inspiratory time and the capacity to increase respiratory rate. Patients with COPD increase their end expiratory lung volumes with exercise in contrast to normal people who reduce end expiratory lung volumes in such circumstances.[10,11]

Table II. Ventilatory limitations in COPD.

a. *Expiratory airflow limitation.*
   Reduced FEV_1, low maximum ventilation;
   Increased tidal volume: inspiratory time ratio
b. *Hyperinflation.*
   Increased functional residual capacity, low maximum inspiratory pressure.
c. *Respiratory muscle strength/endurance.*
   Low maximum inspiratory pressure;
   Reduced maximum sustainable ventilatory capacity.
d. *Increased work of breathing.*
   Increased respiratory rate,
   Increased physiological dead space as a ratio of tidal volume;
   Increased tidal volume: inspiratory time ratio .

Inspiratory muscle strength is diminished in COPD and many neuromuscular disorders due to generalized muscle weakness and fatigue.[12] Ventilatory dead space (V_D) rises[13] increasing the V_D/V_T ratio to cause an increase in ventilatory requirement to eliminate CO_2.

The anaerobic threshold is normal in position but unattainable in severe disease. Work of breathing is increased demanding greater oxygen consumption (VO_2). Overall, the maximum voluntary ventilation (MVV) is reduced and readily attained in exercise.[14] For many patients the maximum exercise ventilation ($V_E$max) = MVV.[15,16] Exercise $V_E$max is normally about 70% of MVV in normal people.[17]

Circulatory Limitation

Patients with respiratory disorders are generally ventilatory rather than circulatory limited but circulatory limitations may be coincidental or occasional consequential. Although pulmonary artery pressure (Ppa) and total pulmonary vascular resistance (TPVR) are raised in COPD and lung fibrosis, they rarely interfere with cardiac output either at rest or on exercise. Except for severely decompensated cor pulmonale patients the right ventricular ejection fraction (RVEF) is relatively normal.[18] Most COPD patients do not have the normal increase in RVEF on exercise and in some it may fall with marked oxygen desaturation.

Although maximum heart rate on exercise is low in COPD it can be increased further if airflow obstruction is reduced by β_2 agonists or O_2 administered to such an extent that a greater workload is achieved (Tab. III).

In contrast in pulmonary vascular disease the hemodynamic stenosis in the pulmonary circulation impairs the ability of the right ventricle to deliver blood to the left atrium at a rate sufficient to meet the demands for an increased cardiac output during exercise.

This inability to increase cardiac output reduces the maximum oxygen consumption, lowers the anaerobic threshold, and alters the VO_2 difference and oxygen pulse in a similar manner to patients with primary heart disease.

Table III. Circulatory limitations in COPD.

---

a. *Pulmonary vascular disease.*
   Increased total pulmonary vascular resistance
   Increased pulmonary artery pressure
   Lowered right ventricular ejection fraction on exercise
   Increased tVO_2
b. *Myocardial contractility.*
c. *Peripheral vascular disease.*

Co-existent coronary artery disease limits the increase in stroke volume and cardiac output during exercise. The consequent poor oxygen delivery to the exercising muscles leads to anaerobic metabolism, lactic acidosis, muscle pain and fatigue.[13,19] Chronic metabolic acidosis occurs even at rest, worsens on exercise and consequently needs a much greater ventilation in an attempt to maintain blood pH homeostasis so exacerbating the ventilatory requirements of COPD.

Peripheral vascular disease prevents vasodilatation which normally allows increased blood supply to working muscles during exercise. Such vasodilatation is essential to increase the transport of oxygen to supply muscles with high and increasing oxygen requirements.[20] When muscle metabolism changes to anaerobic respiratory, lactic acid is partly responsible for pain which may occur at relatively low work rates with severe disease. Lactic acidosis stimulates ventilation through increased CO_2 production and fall in arterial pH, and VO_2 max and the anaerobic threshold are lowered. Severe reduction in muscle perfusion induces systemic lactic acidosis. Exercise is then terminated by claudication rather than by heart rate or ventilatory limitations.

$\dot{V}/\dot{Q}$ Inequality

$\dot{V}/\dot{Q}$ inequality arises from a number of imbalances between ventilation and perfusion (Tab. IV).

In COPD there is an increased ventilatory requirement due to inefficient ventilation of parts of the lung which are still perfused.[21] This leads to an increase in the alveolar arterial PO_2 difference ($D(A-a)O_2$). $D(A-a)O_2$ increases with increasing workload but at different rates in COPD, pulmonary vascular disease and pulmonary fibrosis with resultant fall in SaO_2 on exercise. Likewise arterial end tidal PCO_2 differences ($D(a-ETCO_2)$) are raised and increases at high work rates rather than fall as occurs in normal subjects. In pulmonary vascular disease a good ventilatory reserve is preserved but perfusion to ventilated alveoli is impaired, increasing alveolar dead space and V_D/V_T ratio creating a persistently positive $D(a-ET)CO_2$. Even though pulmonary vascular disease may have a normal PaO_2 at rest,

Table IV. Ventilation/perfusion inequality in COPD.

---

a. *High $\dot{V}/\dot{Q}$ units.*
   Increased dead space to tidal volume ratio;
   Increased Ve/VCO_2;
   Increased $P(a-ET)CO_2$
b. *Low $\dot{V}/\dot{Q}$ units.*
   Increased alveolar-arterial oxygen gradient;
   Fall in oxygen saturation on exercise

---

arterial hypoxemia progressively worsens as work load increases. The time available for diffusion equilibrium for O_2 is shortened by the reduced volume of functional capillary beds.

With exercise pulmonary blood flow increases reducing further the time available for equilibration of alveolar and capillary PO_2. Hypoxemia during exercise is worsened by right to left shunting. This may be through a patent foramen ovale. The high right sided pressures seen in patients with pulmonary hypertension open the foramen inducing right to left cardiac shunts.

Muscular Limitations

Muscular limitations are outlined in table V. Generalized muscle wasting and weakness is a feature of severe emphysema but the cause is not understood.[12] It is often exacerbated by therapy with corticosteroids and disuse of advancing disease. Malnutrition and negative calorie balance may be surprisingly severe but lead to deconditioning of muscle activity, reduced maximal inspiratory and expiratory pressures and mechanical inefficiency.[22-24] Such limitations pose severe exercise limitation in some patients.

Table V. Muscular limitations in COPD.

---

a. *Deconditioning.*
   Increased lactic acid production;
   Reduced CaO_2-$C\bar{v}O_2$;*
   Reduced PO_2
b. *Malnutrition.*
   Reduced maximum inspiratory pressure;
   Reduced maximum expiratory pressure
c. *Mechanical efficiency.*
   Increased Wmus-Wext

---

*CaO_2-$C\bar{v}O_2$:Concentration difference between arterial and mixed venous blood.

Psychological Limitations

In all major diseases, psychological elements affect the manner in which a patient responds to his disease, both in terms of the exercise limitation the patient is prepared to endure against the degree of discomfort he will accept[25] (Tab. VI). Motivation is important. This is not only affected by the personal make-up but also by the speed of disease onset and the ability to adapt to it. These complex personal factors will further be affected by the opinions of close family, society and even

Table VI. Psychological limitations in COPD.

---

a. *Motivation.*
   Increased BR;*
   increased HRR;*
   decreased LA*
b. *Perceived exertion.*
   Increased Borg score
c. *Dyspnea.*
   Increased visual analog score
d. *Confidence, embarrassment, fear.*

---

*BR, breathing rate; HRR, heart rate response; LA, lactic acidosis.

---

their doctors. Self confidence, embarrassment and even fear will each have some input into the patient's willingness to exercise.

They will affect the perception of exertion and the amount of dyspnea produced. All the psychological factors as well as limiting exertional tolerance will also affect the patient's ability to attain a satisfactory level of training and will also influence acceptance of any improvement produced.

Other Factors Limiting Exercise in COPD

Obesity, anemia and cigarette smoking limit exercising capability. Rehabilitation programs must deal with these hurdles to allow the full benefits to be achieved. Obesity demands a greater cardiovascular and respiratory response for any given work rate compared with normal people.[26] Cardiac output is raised even at rest and therefore limits the potential response to exercise. Chest wall obesity and the constraining pressure from the abdomen tend to "strap" the chest.[27]

End expiratory lung volume is low, sometimes at the level of residual volume leading to atelectasis and hypoxemia at rest.[28] Low lung volumes mechanically increase pulmonary vascular resistance.

The increased cost in terms of oxygen requirement for performing mechanical work is predictable, as is the degree of obesity dependent upward displacement of the VO_2 work rate relationship. Although VO_2 max and anaerobic threshold are low in relation to body mass, they are normal in terms of height or lean body mass.[29] Atelectasis improves on exercise with a resultant correction of the hypoxemia. Obese patients should lose weight and exercise as much as possible. In anemia the reduced oxygen carrying capacity leads to a marked reduction in the anaerobic threshold which at very low work rates induces a metabolic acidosis and resultant hyperventilation.

Cigarette smoking affects the blood, the cardiovascular system and the lungs.[30] Carboxyhemoglobin reduces arterial oxygen content and causes a shift of the oxygen dissociation curve to the left.[31] During exercise capillary blood flow may fail to supply adequate oxygen for aerobic metabolism. The anaerobic threshold is lowered. Smoking increases heart rate and blood pressure and aggravates ventilation perfusion mismatching. In the presence of lung disease smoking further increases airways resistance.

Conclusion

In chronic lung disease of whatever type limitation of exercise may be due to a complex of different factors which require detailed evaluation if the rehabilitation is to be effectively directed towards maximum patient response and benefit.

References

1. Casaburi R., Storer T.W., Wasserman K.: Mediation of reduced ventilatory response to exercise after endurance training. J. Appl. Physiol. 1987; 63: 1533-1538
2. Davis J.S., Frank M.H., Whipp B.J., Wasserman K.: Anaerobic threshold alterations caused by endurance training in middle-aged men. J. Appl.Physiol 1979; 46: 1039-1046
3. Ready E.A., Quinney A.H.: Alternations in anaerobic threshold as the result of endurance training and detraining. Med. Sci. Sports Exerc. 1982; 14: 292-296
4. Kumagai S., Nishizumi M., Tanaka K.: Application of lactate threshold to endurance sports science. J. Hum. Ergol. 1987; 16: 129-136
5. Brown H.V., Wasserman K.: Exercise performance in chronic obstructive pulmonary disease. Med. Clin. North. Am. 1981; 65: 525-46
6. Jones N.L., Jones G., Edwards R.H.T.: Exercise tolerance in chronic airway obstruction. Am. Rev. Respir. Dis. 1971; 103: 477-79
7. Sue D.Y., Wasserman K., Moricca R.B. et al. Metabolic acidosis during exercise in patients with chronic obstructive pulmonary disease. Chest 1988;94: 931-938
8. Grimby G., Stiksa J.: Flow-volume curves and breathing patterns during exercise in patients with obstructive lung disease. Scand. J. Clin. Lab. Invest. 1970;25: 303-313
9. Potter W.A., Olafsson S., Hyatt R.E.: Ventilatory mechanics and expiratory flow limitation during exercise in patients with obstructive lung disease. J. Clin. Invest. 1971;50: 910-919
10. Stubbing D.G., Pengelly L.D., Morse J.L. et al. Pulmonary mechanics during exercise in subjects with chronic airflow obstruction. J. Appl. Physiol. 1980;49: 511-515
11. Dodd D.S., Brancatisano T., Engel L.A.: Chest wall mechanics during exercise in patients with severe chronic airflow obstruction. Am. Rev. Respir. Dis.1984; 129: 33-38
12. Rochester D.F., Braun N.M.T.: Determinants of maximal inspiratory pressure in chronic obstructive pulmonary disease. Am. Rev. Respir. Dis. 1985;132: 42-47
13. Nery L.E., Wasserman K., French W., Oren A., Davis J .A.: Contrasting cardiovascular and respiratory responses to exercise in mitral valve and chronic obstructive pulmonary diseases. Chest 1983; 83: 446-53
14. Clark T.J. H., Freedman S., Campbell E. J.M. et al.: The ventilatory capacity of patients with chronic airways obstruction. Clin. Sci. 1969; 36: 307-316

70

15. Mahler D.A., Harver A.: Prediction of peak oxygen consumption in obstructive airway disease. Med. Sci. Sports Exerc. 1988;20: 574-578

16. Matthews J.I., Bush B.A., Ewald F.W.: Exercise responses during incremental and high intensity and low intensity steady state exercise in patients with obstructive lung disease and normal control subjects. Chest 1989;96: 11-17

17. Jones N.L.: Pulmonary gas exchange during exercise in patients with chronic airway obstruction. Clin. Sci. 1966; 31: 3950

18. Macnee W.: Right ventricular function in cor pulmonale. Cardiology 1988; 75, Sl, 30-40

19. Rubin S.A., Brown H.V.: Ventilation and gas exchange during exercise in severe chronic heart failure. Am. Rev. Respir. Dis. 1984; 129 (Suppl): S63-S64

20. Bylund-Fellenius A.C., Walker P.M., Elander A., Schersten T.: Peripheral vascular disease. Am. Rev. Respir. Dis. 1984; 129 (Suppl): S65-S67

21. Wasserman K., Hansen J. E. et al.: Pathophysiology of disorders limiting exercise. Chapter 4: *Principles of Exercise Testing.* Philadelphia, Lea and Febinger, 1987

22. Servera E., Gimenez M., Mohan-Kumar T. et al.: Oxygen uptake at maximal exercises in chronic airflow obstruction. Bull. Eur. Physiopathol. Respir. 1983; 19: 553-556

23. Allard C., Jones N.L., Killian K. J.: Static peripheral skeletal muscle strength and exercise capacity in patients with chronic airflow limitation. Am. Rev. Respir. Dis. 1989; 139: A90

24. Gallagher C.G., Younes M.: Breathing pattern during and after maximal exercise in patients with chronic obstructive lung disease, interstitial lung disease and cardiac disease, and in normal subjects. Am. Rev. Respir. Dis. 1986; 133: 581-586

25. Borg G.A.V.: Psychophysical bases of perceived exertion. Med. Sci. Sports Exerc. 1982; 14: 377-381

26. Alexander J.K., Amad K.H., Cole V.W.: Observations on some clinical features of extreme obesity, with particular reference to circulatory effect. Am. J. Med. 1962; 32: 512-524

27. Gilbert R., Sipple J.H., Auchincloss J.H.: Respiratory control and work of breathing in obese subjects. J. Appl. Physiol. 1961; 16: 21-26

28. Ray C.S., Sue D.Y., Bray G., Hansen J.E., Wasserman K.: Effects of obesity on respiratory function. Am. Rev. Respir. Dis. 1983; 128(3): 501-506

29. Buskirk E., Taylor H.L.: Maximal oxygen intake and its relation to body composition, with special reference to chronic physical activity and obesity. J. Appl. Physiol. 1957; 11: 72-78

30. Pirnay S., Dujardin J., Deroanne R., Petit J.M.: Muscular exercise during intoxication by carbon monoxide. J. Appl. Physiol. 1971; 31: 573-575

31. Vogel J.A., Gleser M.A.: Effect of carbon monoxide on oxygen transport during exercise. J. Appl. Physiol. 1972; 32: 234-239

32. Hirsch G.L., Sue D.Y., Wasserman K., Robinson T.E., Hansen J.E.: Immediate effects of cigarette smoking on the cardiorespiratory responses to exercise. J. Appl. Physiol. 1985;58: 1975-1981

8. Exercise in Chronic Obstructive Disease: Adaptation to Exercise and Practical Indices

R. SERGYSELS, A. SANNA, A. LACHMAN

Clinique de Pneumologie, Hôpital Universitaire Saint-Pierre, Bruxelles, Belgium

Adaptation to Exercise

A limited exercise capacity is the prime feature of chronic airflow obstruction and results mostly from pulmonary limitation, especially related to the abnormal mechanical characteristics of the respiratory system.[1]

Respiratory drive and breathing pattern

When compared to normals, patients with chronic obstructive disease (COPD) show at the same oxygen uptake (VO_2) rapid shallow breathing (RSB), i.e. lower tidal volume (VT), higher breathing frequency (BF) with shorter inspiratory (TI) and expiratory (TE) time. The duty cycle (TI/TTOT) is usually found to be similar to that in normal subjects,[2] except if bronchospasm occurs during exercise which leads to severe expiratory flow limitation and increased TE.[3]

Despite impeded ventilation (VE), higher occlusion pressure at the mouth (p=0.1) and the increase of mean inspiratory flow (VT/TI), indicate increased respiratory drive in COPD (Fig. 1) with and without hypercapnia.[2]

RSB and increased respiratory drive result probably from the mechanical adaptation to increased impedance of the respiratory system, and from central mechanisms integrating reflexes originating from chemoreceptors and from the lung and/or the chest wall.[2,4]

Lung and chest wall mechanics

During exercise but even at rest, COPD patients may reach maximal expiratory flow despite a progressive increase in the end-expiratory volume during exercise (FRC). Expiratory flow limitation results from increasing expiratory air-flow resistances (Raw) and from loss of lung elastic recoil.[5,6]

Thus, an increase in VE during exercise is usually achieved by an increase in end-expiratory volumes to improve expiratory flow developed in the effort dependent part of the flow volume curve (Fig.2).[5]

However, this hyperinflation is associated with an expansion of the rib cage and therefore inspiratory muscles are located on their pressure-volume relationship where both the diaphragm (that became flatter) and the other inspiratory muscles are working inefficiently.[7] Thus the inspiratory muscles have to develop high pressures, probably close to the maximal pressures they may generate, and these muscles may eventually become fatigued.[8]

The increased work of breathing may also be due to the expiratory muscles recruitment.[9] Compensatory mechanisms may exist: active expiration with decreased abdominal volume at end expiration and fast relaxation of the abdominal wall at the beginning of inspiration may give a better length-tension relationship of the diaphragm and a fast caudal displacement of this muscle, without important mechanical work for this muscle.[10-12]

Finally, in undernourished COPD patients, the weak respiratory muscles (resulting from their reduced mass and thickness) may further decrease the performance of the respiratory pump.[13,14]

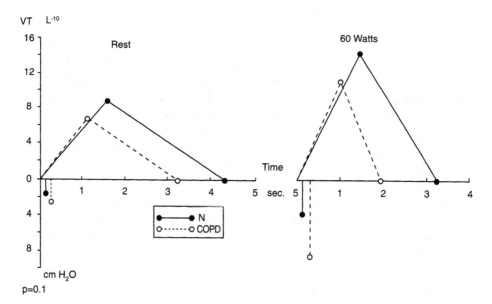

Fig. 1. Comparison at rest and at 60 watts of the breathing pattern and occlusion pressure (p= 0.1) in normals and in patients affected by COPD.

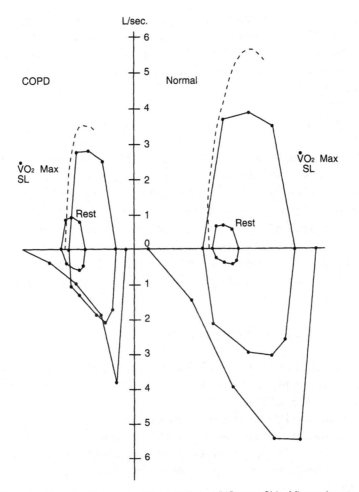

Fig. 2. Comparison at rest and at the maximal load achieved (VO_2 max SL) of flow volume curves in normals and in patients affected by COPD. Maximal flow volumes are also presented for both groups.

Gas exchange problems

During exercise, the changes in arterial partial pressures of O_2 and CO_2 (PaO_2, $PaCO_2$) are variable, depending on the type of the clinical syndrome and on the severity of airway obstruction.[4,15]

Usually exercise induced hypoxia is found in patients with emphysema, severe pulmonary hypertension (PHT) and a low PaO_2 at rest.[16]

When $PaCO_2$ is found to increase during exercise, it may be explained either by ventilatory limitation or by wasted ventilation due to alveolar hypoventilation observed with RSB, that increases dead space tidal volume ratio (VD/VT).[2,16]

Although in most patients at the beginning of exercise alveolar to arterial PO_2 difference $P(a/A)CO_2$ increases and arterial to end-tidal PCO_2 difference $P(a/A)CO_2$ decreases these parameters that reflect V/Q matching and VD/VT ratio can remain stable during incremental exercise, showing an acceptable capacity for gas exchange control.[3,4]

Cardiac performance

In COPD patients, the heart rate/oxygen uptake relationship (VO_2/HR) is lower than in normals but the slope until maximal O_2 uptake (VO_2 max) is usually found to be normal. This finding, and a large heart rate reserve (HRR), may indicate that left ventricular function probably remains normal in stable COPD patients.[3]

However in patients experiencing hypoxia at rest and during exercise, the main cardiac characteristic is right ventricular hypertrophy due to pulmonary hypertension.[17] The right ventricular ejection fraction (RVEF) measured at exercise shows no increase when the clinical signs and symptoms of cor pulmonale are beginning to appear.[18]

Exercise Strategies and Practical Indices

Exercise testing evaluation is difficult because various investigators use a variety of protocols probably due to a lack of recommended guidelines for exercise testing in normals and in patients.

However, most laboratories in Europe use a bicycle ergometer and study patients with a continuous increase in load with a maximal exercise period of 8 to 12 minutes.In clinical practice, most patients stop exercising below a true maximal oxygen consumption and complain about symptoms such as dyspnea, exhaustion or leg pain.

Therefore the maximal VO_2 measured is called the maximal O_2 consumption limited by the symptoms (VO_2 max SL). But as predicted values for VO_2 do not apply to such patients, a variety of other indices have been proposed for evaluation of the patients.[19,20]

The most useful seem to be the evaluation of cardiac or respiratory reserves,[20] the anaerobic threshold (AT) level[21] and the evaluation of dyspnea.[22] Other indices derived from EKG, ear oxymetry, blood pressure, oxygen pulse, VD/VT, blood gas analysis, pulmonary pressure, etc. may be helpful for a more precise analysis.

Practical Indices at Maximal Exercise Level (VO₂ max SL)

It is important to appreciate the exercise limiting factors. Is the patient limited by poor ventilatory reserve, by poor cardiac adaptation or both?

Ventilatory limitation is usually appreciated by expressing the ventilation achieved at maximal level of exercise as a percentage of the direct or more easily the indirect maximal voluntary ventilation (MVV) (for instance FEV_1 x 36).[23]

Normals or cardiac patients usually have a ventilatory reserve of about 30% whereas in COPD patients VE max/MVV reaches 100% or even more.

Cardiac limitation is appreciated by the heart rate reserve (HRR) which reaches a maximal value at a relatively late work rate, or better by the O_2 pulse which is reduced when the cardiac stroke volume is decreased.[20] We have to keep in mind that O_2 pulse will also be low when anemia, high levels of carbohemoglobin or severe arterial hypoxemia are present.

Practical indices at submaximal level

It is often important to examine the evolution of the variables at submaximal exercise, especially since many patients will stop exercising well below the expected maximum values. Some indices may be used to decide whether the variables are abnormal at a given level of exercise, thus registering impairment of specific mechanisms.

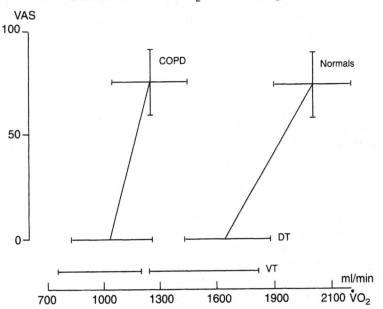

Fig. 3. Comparison of dyspnea sensation during an incremental protocol in normals and in patients affected by COPD. A dyspneic threshold (DT) is found to be close to the ventilatory threshold (VT). The O_2 level for DT and VT is obviously higher in normals.

One of the most useful parameters is the anaerobic threshold.

Wasserman et al. clearly defined noninvasive ways to determine this exercise level.[20] In our experience, by analyzing the VE/VO_2 and VCO_2/VO_2 relationships, we were able to locate a ventilatory threshold well correlated with the lactate threshold.[24]

The AT level is helpful for the differential diagnosis of cardiorespiratory disorders. Conditions that limit O_2 flow to the exercising muscles during exercise will most likely cause the AT to be low. Combined with the previous parameters, the pathophysiology of exercise limitation can be further subclassified. Several authors proposed useful algorithms through a logical procedure for differential diagnosis with exercise-derived data.[20,25]

Measuring dyspnea during exercise

One of the absolute indications for exercise testing is to quantify and elucidate the mechanism contributing to dyspnea. This measure is usually appreciated by psychophysical methods such as the *Borg Scale* or the *Visual Analog Scale*.[22]

In our experince, both COPD patients and normal subjects show a dyspneic threshold and we found a quasi-linear increase in the sensation above this level. Furthermore, the dyspneic threshold seems to be close to the ventilatory threshold and is influenced by the breathing pattern (VT, VT/TI, TI/TTOT, BF), emphasizing the role of the ventilatory demand and the breathing pattern during exercise in the genesis of dyspnea (Fig. 3).[24]

References

1. Brown H.V., Wasserman K.: Exercise performance in chronic obstructive pulmonary disease. Bull. Eur. Physiopath. Respir. 1977; 13: 409-413
2. Van Meerhaeghe A., Sergysels R.: Control of breathing during exercise in patients with chronic airflow limitation with or without hypercapnia. Chest 1983; 84: 565-570
3. Nery L.E., Wasserman K., French W., Oren A., Davis J.A.: Contrasting cardiovascular and respiratory responses to exercise in mitral valve and chronic obstructive pulmonary disease. Chest 1983; 83: 446-453
4. Jones N.L., Berman L.B.: Gas exchange in chronic airflow obstruction. Am. Rev. Respir. Dis. 1984; 129: (suppl.) S81-S83
5. Potter W.A., Olefsson S., Hyatt R.E.: Ventilatory mechanics and expiratory flow limitation during exercise in patients with obstructive lung disease. J. Clin. Invest. 1971; 50: 310-313
6. Stubbing D.G., Pengelly L.D., Morse S.L.C., Jones N.: Pulmonary mechanics during exercise in subjects with chronic airflow obstruction. J. Appl. Physiol. 1980; 49: 511-515
7. Pengelly L.D., Alderson A.M., Milic-Emili J.: Mechanics of the diaphragm. J. Appl. Physiol. 1971; 30: 797-805
8. Grassino A., Gross D., Macklem P.T., Roussos C.H., Zagelbaum G.: Inspiratory muscle fatigue as a factor limiting exercise. Bull. Eur. Physiopath. Respir. 1979; 15: 105-111

9. Dodd D.S., Yarom J., Loring S.H., Engel L.A.: O$_2$ cost of inspiratory and expiratory resistive breathing in humans. J. Appl. Physiol. 1988; 65: 2518-2523

10. Dodd D.S., Brancatisano T., Engel L.A., Chest wall mechanics during exercise in patients with severe chronic airflow obstruction. Am. Rev. Respir. Dis. 1984; 129; 33-38

11. Dodd D.R., Brancatisano T.P., Engel L.A.: Effect of abdominal strapping on chest wall mechanics during exercise in patients with severe air-flow obstruction. Am. Rev. Respir. Dis. 1985; 131: 816-821

12. Erpicum B., Willeput R., Sergysels R., De Coster A.: Does abdominal breathing below FRC gives a mechanical support for inspiration? Clin. Respir. Physiol. 1984; 20: 20a (abstract)

13. Arora N.S., Rochester D.F.: COPD and human diaphragm muscle dimensions. Chest 1987; 91: 719-724

14. Rochester D.F., Brown N.T.M., Arora N.S.: Respiratory muscle strength in chronic obstructive pulmonary disease. Am. Rev. Respir. Dis. 1979; 119: 151-154

15. Raffestin B., Escourrou P., Legrand A. et al.: Circulatory transport of oxygen in patients with chronic airflow obstruction exercising maximally. Am. Rev. Respir. Dis. 1982; 125: 426-431

16. Dantzker D.R., D'Alonzo E.G.: The effect of exercise on pulmonary gas exchange in patients with severe chronic obstructive disease. Am. Rev. Respir. Dis. 1986; 134: 1135-1139

17. Loke S., Mahler D.A., Paul Man S.F., Weidemann H.P., Matthay R.A.: Exercise impairment in chronic obstructive pulmonary disease. Clinics in Chest Medicine 1984; 5: 121-143

18. France A.J., Prescott R.J., Biernacki W., Muir A.L., Maruee W.: Does right ventricular function predict survival in patients with chronic obstructive lung disease? Thorax 1988; 43: 621-626

19. Jones N.L.: *Clinical Exercise Testing*. Philadelphia, Saunders, 1988; 325

20. Wasserman K., Hansen J.E., Sue D.Y., Whipp B.J.: *Principles of Exercise Testing and Interpretation*. Philadelphia, Lea & Febiger, 1987; 274

21. Sue D.Y., Wasserman K., Moricca R.B., Casaburi R.: Metabolic acidosis during exercise in patients with chronic obstructive pulmonary disease. Chest 1988; 94: 931-938

22. Killian K.J.: Dyspnea and exercise. Ann. Rev. Physiol. 1983; 45: 465-479

23. Gandevia B.: Terminology for measurements of ventilatory capacity. Thorax 1957; 12: 290-293

24. Lachman A., Sanna A., Sergysels R.: Use of a visual analog scale at exercise in normals and COPD. International meeting on respiratory muscle fatigue. Florence, Fisioray Editore, Monte Oriolo, 1990; 44

25. Eschenbacher W.L.: An algorithm for the interpretation of cardiopulmonary exercise tests. Chest 1990; 97: 263-267

9. Noninvasive Assessment of Pulmonary Arterial Pressure with Ultrasound

R.TRAMARIN,[1] A.TORBICKI,[2] G.FORNI,[1] M.FRANCHINI[1]

1. *Division of Cardiology, Fondazione Clinica del Lavoro, Care and Research Institute, Montescano, Pavia , Italy*
2. *Department of Hypertension and Angiology, Academy of Medicine, Warszawa, Poland*

Introduction

Noninvasive assessment of pulmonary arterial pressure (PAP) has been attempted for years. However, isolated reports on high correlation between direct pressure measurements and results obtained with noninvasive techniques have not been confirmed in the clinical setting. With the revolution in noninvasive cardiac diagnosis caused by echocardiography, new methods for assessment of pulmonary circulation have been announced over the past fifteen years. Ultrasound examination provided information on morphological and functional effects of pulmonary hypertension. Recently, pressure gradients between selected heart chambers have been successfully estimated with Doppler echocardiography and used for assessment of pulmonary arterial pressures. This paper will critically review currently available ultrasonic methods of potential clinical importance for evaluation of pulmonary hypertension.

Morphological Changes within the Right Heart

Chronic pulmonary hypertension is followed by hypertrophy of the right ventricular free wall. Echocardiographic measurements of the thickness of the right ventricular (RV) free wall have been reported to correlate with results obtained at autopsy.[1] With the introduction of the subcostal approach these methods were available also for a large fraction of patients with cor pulmonale and lung hyperinflation.[2-4] The correlation between right ventricular wall thickness estimated by echocardiography and directly measured PAP was rather poor.[3,4] These findings may in part be explained by low reproducibility of echocadiographic measurements concerning right ventricular wall thickness and mass, related to heavy trabeculation and complex shape of the right ventricle.[5]

Right ventricular diastolic diameter (RVEDD) as an isolated measurement or as an index considering body surface area or left ventricular end-diastolic dimensions (LVEDD) was reported to correlate with mean PAP in patients with chronic obstructive pulmonary disease[3,4,6] but not in patients with mitral stenosis.[7] Acute pulmonary embolism and atrial septal defect are among typical causes of marked increase in the RVEDD/LVEDD ratio.[8,9] In these clinical conditions, however, high RVEDD/LVEDD ratio reflects either the degree of right ventricular failure or the degree of volume overload, rather than the severity of pulmonary hypertension. Right ventricular diastolic dimensions are also increased in patients with previous episodes of right heart failure.[3] Thus, the presence of shunts, important right heart valvular insufficiency or right ventricular failure should be excluded if increased RVEDD is to be considered a marker of pulmonary hypertension. Despite these limitations, RVEDD, preferably compared with LVEDD, is a useful screening test for right ventricular overload, the characteristics of which should further be clarified with other methods.

In contrast to right ventricular dimensions, the diameter of the pulmonary artery or its major branches is not influenced by increased right ventricular diastolic pressure. Correlation was reported between pulmonary artery (RPA) diameter measured by M-mode echo from the suprasternal approach and PAP in patients with chronic pulmonary hypertension.[10] Although the right pulmonary artery was dilated in 78% of patients with acute pulmonary embolism, no correlation with pulmonary arterial pressure was found (Ref. 9 and personal communication). In patients with increased pulmonary flow due to left to right shunt, dilatation of the RPA reflects both chronic increase in stroke volume and pulmonary arterial pressure. The diameter of the main pulmonary artery measured from the subcostal or parasternal approach was not found useful for assessment of pulmonary arterial pressure in a multicentre study of patients with chronic lung diseases.[11]

Some authors reported that in patients with chronic lung disease it is possible to deduce the mean pulmonary artery pressure (PAMP) using multivariate regressions based on measurements of RVEDD, LVEDD, diameter of the tricuspid annulus and right ventricular free wall thickness. However, these observations were not confirmed by others.[3,4]

Functional Changes in the Right Heart

The position and motion pattern of the intraventricular septum was found useful in differential diagnosis of right ventricular dilatation.[12,13] In pure right ventricular pressure overload the displacement of the septum towards the left ventricular cavity

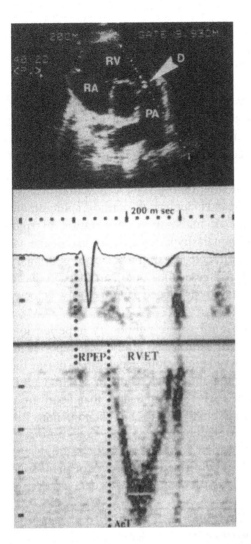

Fig. 1 Pulsed wave Doppler assessment of right ventricular systolic events. *Upper panel:* pulsed wave Doppler sample volume (D) in the right ventricular outflow tract (RA: right atrium; RV: right ventricle; PA: main pulmonary artery). *Lower panel:* measurements obtained from pulsed wave Doppler tracing (RPEP: right ventricular preejection period; RVET: right ventricular ejection time. AcT: acceleration time of right ventricular ejection).

is more pronounced at end-systole. However, in some patients with moderate compensated pulmonary hypertension the pattern of diastolic septal bulging towards the left ventricle was described.[14-16]

Response of the right ventricle to increased afterload is that of prolongation of right ventricular preejection period (RPEP), shortening of right ventricular ejection time (RVET) and decrease of RV ejection fraction.[17,18] The measurements of systolic time intervals can be reliably performed either by M-mode or by Doppler echocardiography (Fig. 1).[19]

The Doppler method yields a higher success rate even in patients with lung hyperinflation, who are particularly difficult to study by ultrasound.[20] Boyd reported on high accuracy of prediction of pulmonary arterial diastolic pressure (PADP) with right ventricular isovolumic contraction time (RVICT) measured by M-mode echocardiography (r=0.92, SEE = 3.0 mmHg) in 17 patients with chronic cor pulmonale.[21] A later study, however, could not confirm these excellent results.[16] Unfortunately, RV systolic time intervals and ejection fraction are affected by RV preload, contractility, interventricular conduction defects, heart rate, and the presence of tricuspid insufficiency. Despite an initial report[22] RV ejection fraction is moreover very difficult to assess with echocardiography because of the complex right ventricular shape.[5]

Among systolic events, the pattern of flow during right ventricular ejection received most attention. M-mode, contrast and Doppler echocardiographic studies independently reported on the presence of midsystolic deceleration of right ventricular ejection in patients with pulmonary hypertension. By use of the M-mode technique this was evidenced by partial closure of the posterior pulmonary valve leaflet,[23] in echo-contrast studies by changes in the slope of artifacts produced by gas microbubbles[24] and in Doppler studies by a notched pattern of flow velocity in the right ventricular outflow tract.[25]

These findings were considered specific for severe pulmonary hypertension. Only idiopathic dilatation of the proximal pulmonary artery was reported to produce a similar phenomenon.[26] We observed midsystolic deceleration during the inspiratory phase also in patients with acute pulmonary embolism or with COPD despite normal or only mildly elevated PAP. This indicates that apart from pulmonary hypertension other factors may contribute to this phenomenon. Recently, Turkevich et al.[27] reported a correlation between PAP and timing of midsystolic deceleration which occurred earlier with increasing pressure. Using high fidelity pressure transducers the authors confirmed the presence of an inverted pressure gradient across the pulmonary valve coinciding with deceleration of forward pulmonary flow.

The exact timing of peak systolic velocity within the RV outflow tract measured with respect to the beginning of forward systolic flow (acceleration time, AcT) with pulsed wave Doppler echocardiography allowed for qualitative analysis of the RV ejection pattern (Fig. 1).[25] It was feasible in 70 to 97% of patients, including those with hyperinflation of the lungs, in whom the subcostal approach provided a convenient way to examine the right ventricular outflow tract.[20,28,29] The reported correlation coefficients with PAP varied from r= –0.65 to –0.91, depending mostly on the range of pulmonary arterial pressure studied.[20,28-34] It was pointed out that the regression equations suggested by different authors prevented their general application.[35] This was partly due to lack of agreement as to whether the right ventricular outflow tract or the main pulmonary artery should be used for flow velocity registrations,[36,37] and whether measurements should be corrected for cardiac output,[32,38] heart rate, RVET or RPEP.

The mechanism relating AcT to pressure within the pulmonary artery remains unclear. Velocity of the pressure wave within the pulmonary vessels is increased in pulmonary hypertension. Thus, reflected pressure waves reappear earlier within the main pulmonary artery opposing the driving force of the right ventricular ejection. In fact, age independently decreased AcT in a population of patients with cor pulmonale (personal observation), probably affecting the elastic properties of proximal pulmonary arteries. In addition, changes in right ventricular contractility were recently reported to influence AcT.[39] Whatever the mechanism and whatever the population studied AcT was found to estimate the mean PAP with standard error of not less than 6 to 9 mmHg. Although the potential of monitoring the acute or chronic changes of PAP using measurements of AcT has not been proven, preliminary reports are discouraging.[41,19]

Among diastolic events used for prediction of PAP M-mode echocardiography analyzed diastolic motion of the point of coaption of the pulmonary valve (e-f slope, atrial wave). Flat e-f slope and absent atrial wave considered markers of pulmonary hypertension.[23,42] Later it was found that these findings were predominantly due to decreased emptying rate of the left atrium in patients with mitral stenosis and quantitative evaluation of pulmonary valve echogram was abandoned.[43,44] The nomogram describing relation of the right ventricular relaxation time (RVIRT) to pulmonary artery systolic pressure and heart rate was based on mechanocardiographic findings,[45] but was reported useful also in M-mode and Doppler measurements.[46,47] The mechanism of prolongation of isovolumic relaxation is more complex than initially suggested by Burstin, who assumed a constant rate of RV early diastolic pressure decline regardless of peak systolic pressure. Also Burstin's nomogram was found to overestimate the influence of heart rate on isovolumic relaxation.[48] Apart from pressure, right ventricular relaxation is probably affected by other factors, such as hypertrophy, fibrosis and ischemia. Nevertheless, correlation coefficients with systolic pulmonary arterial pressure were in the range of 0.66-0.97 with SEE of 6-9 mmHg.[20,46,47,49] The changes in pulmonary artery pressure were reflected by respective changes in relaxation time.[46] The major drawback of both M-mode and Doppler measurements of RVIRT is in non-simultaneous assessment of the pulmonary and tricuspid valvular events, precluding the use of this method in patients with atrial fibrillation.[49] In patients with chronic cor pulmonale, free of arrhythmias, right ventricular isovolumic relaxation time could be evaluated with M-mode in 30% and with Doppler in about 80% of cases.[16,20]

Pressure Gradients within the Right Heart

Continuous wave Doppler combined with two-dimensional echocardiography provides an excellent method to assess high velocity jets within the heart. The velocity of the jet is in turn directly related to the pressure difference up- and

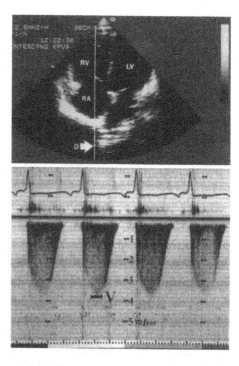

Fig. 2. Assessment of retrograde tricuspid valve systolic gradient with continuous wave Doppler. *Upper panel:* reference line of continuous wave Doppler (D) displayed on two-dimensional echocardiographic image (RA: right atrium; RV right ventricle; LV: left ventricle). *Lower panel:* jet of tricuspid valve regurgitation recorded with continuous wave Doppler (V: max velocity of jet used for calculation of tricuspid gradient, according to the Bernoulli equation: P1–P2 = 4V². In this case: V= 3.8 m/s. Thus, the gradient is calculated as: 4 x 14.4 = 57.6 mmHg).

downstream. This relation is described by the equation of Bernoulli. For hemodynamic purposes the simplified Bernoulli equation has gained broad acceptance. It permits one to calculate the pressure gradient at the origin of a jet by multiplying the second power of the maximal jet velocity by four (P1–P2 = 4 V max^2)(Fig. 2). Even trivial tricuspid valve regurgitation, often found with Doppler both in normals and patients (Tab. I), permits noninvasive assessment of systolic retrograde gradient between right ventricle and right atrium. When a Doppler study is performed simultaneously with right heart catheterization it shows perfect, beat to beat agreement with the results of direct pressure gradient measurements.[50]

The correlation coefficient between Doppler and direct pressure assessment of retrograde systolic tricuspid valve gradient in patients with postcapillary pulmonary hypertension or intracardiac shunts was 0.96-0.97 with SEE 4.9-7 mmHg.[50-52] Right ventricular outflow tract obstruction must be excluded and right atrial pressure should be added to the retrograde systolic tricuspid gradient if it is used for calculation of systolic pulmonary arterial pressure.

The assumed value for right atrial pressure may represent a source of error as the accuracy of its estimates based on echographic measurements of the vena cava or right atrium is not accurate sufficient.[7,53]

Recently, assessment of dynamic changes in IVC diameter during controlled obstructed inspiration (sonospirometry) was reported to yield good correlations

Table I. Prevalence of tricuspid valve regurgitation (TVR) with continuous wave Doppler echocardiography.

Reported by	Population studied	Prevalence of TVR, n/N (%)	Measurable peak jet velocity, n/N
Michelsen et al.[60]	Healthy women	31/95	?
Yock and Popp[61]	Patients with clinical signs of pulmonary hypertension	56/62	54/62
Berger et al.[51]	Patients with bedside Swan-Ganz monitoring	41/69 (59%)*	?
Currie et al.[50]	Patients submitted to left heart cath	54/64 (84%)	48/64 (75%)
Torbicki et al.[20]	Patients with chronic lung disease	32/70 (46%)	17/70 (24%)

* The prevalence of tricuspid valve regurgitation strongly depends on presence and severity of pulmonary hypertension. n: the number of patients in whom valvular regurgitation was found (or its velocity could be measured) using Doppler echocardiography. N: the total number of patients studied with Doppler echocardiography.

with right atrial pressure, but the method required special equipment and was time consuming.[54] Besides, evaluation of the jugular veins did not improve accuracy of noninvasive prediction of PASP when compared to arbitrarily assumed right atrial pressure of 10 mmHg (r = 0.90 vs. 0.89 and SEE for both methods 8 mmHg.[50] Calculations of PASP based on velocity of tricuspid regurgitation are limited to jets angulated with the ultrasound beam by less than 20°, larger angles producing important underestimation of the velocity with CW Doppler.

The major limitation of the method in patients with cor pulmonale is in the low prevalence of tricuspid jets suitable for measurements.[11,20,55]

Recently, intravenous injection of agitated saline was successfully used to increase the percent of good-quality recordings of tricuspid jet velocity also in patients with COPD.[56,57]

Respiration, if not taken into account, may influence the accuracy of pressure estimations. If the clear spectral outline can be recorded only at inspiration, the jet velocity is higher, probably due to a Starling effect induced by enhanced venous return. Thus, in some patients Doppler data obtained only from inspiratory beats are compared to directly measured pressures, averaged throughout the whole respiratory cycle. The percent of patients which could be studied increases, but the accuracy of estimation falls.

"Color coded" two-dimensional pulsed wave Doppler assistance may improve identification of the jets suitable for assessment of retrograde tricuspid gradients.

Angle correction, even based on "color Doppler" findings, should be discouraged, as it may introduce the possibility of overestimation of PAP. The same applies to the assessment of diastolic pulmonary arterial pressure derived from Doppler measurements of velocity of the jet of pulmonary regurgitation. This method is based on the same Bernoulli principle which was presented earlier in this section.

The velocity of the jet of pulmonary insufficiency, measured at the end of diastole, permits one to calculate the end-diastolic pressure difference between the main pulmonary artery and the right ventricle. Similarly to the tricuspid jet method, right ventricular end-diastolic pressure must be added to the calculated pressure gradient in order to give the estimate of pulmonary artery diastolic pressure. Masuyama reported on excellent results of such an approach (r vs. PADP = 0.92, SEE = 3 mmHg). High prevalence of pulmonary valve regurgitation was reported in several studies (Tab. II). In our experience the method applies to less than 30% of patients, despite color coded two-dimensional Doppler assistance.

The newly introduced trans-esophageal echocardiographic approach does not increase the number of patients who may benefit from noninvasive evaluation of pulmonary arterial pressures based on Doppler assessment of pulmonary and tricuspid retrograde gradients.

The right ventricular outflow tract can be scanned only in cross-sectional planes and the jet of pulmonary regurgitation is usually missed. The axis of the tricuspid valve is usually not parallel to the Doppler beam transmitted from the esophagus, and thus only aberrant jets directed versus the lower portion of the interatrial septum can be considered for velocity measurements (personal observation).

The simplified Bernoulli equation can also be used to calculate the systolic pressure difference between both ventricles in the presence of interventricular septal defect. If obstruction of outflow tract of both ventricles is excluded, the

Table II. Prevalence of pulmonary valve regurgitation (PVR) with continuous wave Doppler echocardiography.

Reported by	Population studied	Prevalence of TVR, n/N (%)	Measurable peak jet velocity, n/N
Yok et al.[61]	Healthy adults	(40%)	?
Michelsen et al.[60]	Healthy women	21/95 (22%)	?
Takao et al.[62]	Healthy women	39/50 (78%)	?
Masuyama et al.[63]	Patients submitted to left heart cath	?	31/45 (69%)
Torbicki et al.[20]	Patients with chronic lung disease	15/70 (21%)	7/70 (10%)

Abbreviations: see Table I.

systolic pulmonary arterial pressure may be calculated by subtraction of the interventricular pressure gradient from systemic systolic pressure.[58,59] Special care must be taken not to over-estimate right sided pressure by measuring significantly angulated jets. In small muscular defects, when blood traverses a relatively long muscular tunnel, the simplified Bernoulli equation should not be applied.[59]

Conclusions

Ultrasound techniques offer several approaches to noninvasive assessment of pulmonary arterial pressures (Tabb. III and IV). None of them is fully reliable. The evaluation of the velocity of retrograde valvular jets within the right heart is a most straightforward method, allowing for reasonable quantitative assessment of pulmonary hypertension, and thus should be applied as a method of choice whenever possible. The method requires the presence of valvular insufficiency and the assumption of right heart diastolic pressures. Short acceleration time of flow

Table III. Comparison of Doppler methods used for assessment of pulmonary arterial pressure: population of a cardiologic department. [50]

Method used	Success rate	Correlation coefficient (r) vs	SEE
TVR jet velocity	72%	0.89 vs PASP	7.4 mmHg
AcT	88%	-0.66 vs PAPM	10 mmHg
(AcT*)	(52%)		(7 mmHg)
RVIRT	64	- vs PASP	-
(RVIRT*)	(22%)		(11 mmHg)

TVR: tricuspid valve regurgitation; AcT: acceleration time of right ventricular ejection; RVIRT: right ventricular isovolumic relaxation time; *: patients with heart rate between 60 and 100 bpm; **: patients without arrhythmias; PAMP: mean pulmonary arterial pressure; PASP: systolic pulmonary arterial pressure.

Table IV. Comparison of Doppler methods used for assessment of pulmonary arterial pressure: population of a pneumologic department.[20]

Method used	Success rate	Correlation coefficient (r) vs	SEE
TVR jet velocity	25%	0.91 vs PASP	7.9 mmHg
AcT	97%	-0.72 vs PMAP	8.3 mmHg
RVIRT**	84%	0.66 vs PASP	11.6 mmHg

Abbreviations: see Table III.

88

velocity in the right ventricular outflow tract (AcT < 80 ms) especially accompanied by midsystolic deceleration occurring throughout the respiratory cycle is strong evidence of pulmonary hypertension. Acceleration time in the range of 80 - 120 ms should be considered a gray zone and qualitative conclusions of clinical importance should be avoided. Long AcT (>120ms) is virtually diagnostic of normal pulmonary arterial pressure. If high speed (100 mm/s) good quality registrations of Doppler tracings of both pulmonary and tricuspid valve flow or leaflet motion are available, Burstin's nomogram may be used for estimation of pulmonary arterial pressure, although calculation of the laboratory's own regression equation should be advised. The information provided by two-dimensional echocardiography on morphologic consequences of pulmonary hypertension should not be missed.

Considered together, ultrasound methods permit one to identify patients with moderate and severe pulmonary hypertension. The accuracy of the echocardiographic method used should always be confronted with the error of pressure estimation which may be accepted in a particular clinical situation. Exact assessment of pulmonary hemodynamics when necessary for important therapeutic decisions should still in most cases rely on right heart catheterization.

References

1. Prakash R., Matsukubo H.: Usefulness of echocardiographic right ventricular measurements in estimating right ventricular hypertrophy and right ventricular pressure. Am. J. Cardiol. 1983; 51: 1036
2. Bertoli L., Rizzato G., Sala G., Merlini R., Lo Cicero S., Pezzano A.: Echocardiographic and hemodynamic assessment of right heart impairment in chronic obstructive lung disease. Respiration 1983; 44: 282
3. Danchin N., Cornette A., Henriquez A., Godenir J.P., Ethevenot G., Polu J.M., Sadoul P.: Two dimensional echocardiographic assessment of the right ventricle in patients with obstructive lung disease. Chest 1987; 92: 229
4. Zenker G., Forche G., Harnouncourt K.: Two-dimensional echocardiography using a subcostal approach in patients with COPD. Chest 1985; 88: 722
5. Foale R., Nihojannopoulos P., McKenna W., Klienebenne A., Nadazdin A., Rowland E., Smith G.: Echocardiographic measurement of the normal adult right ventricle. Br. Heart J. 1986; 56: 33
6. Oswald-Mammosser M., Thierry O., Nyankiye, Dickele M.C., Grange D., Weitzenblum E.: Non-invasive diagnosis of pulmonary hypertension in chronic obstructive pulmonary disease: Comparison of ECG, radiological measurements, echocardiography and myocardial scintigraphy. Eur. J. Respir. Dis. 1984; 73: 646
7. Lambertz H., Krebs W., Soeding S., Wohltmann D., Sechtem U., Kemmer H.P.: Größenbestimmung des rechten Vorhofes bei Patienten mit pulmonaler Hypertonie mittels zweidimensionaler Echokardiographie. Z. Kardiol. 1984; 73: 646
8. Goldberg S.J., Allen H.D., Sahn D.J.: *Pediatric and Adolescent Echocardiography*. Chicago, Year Book Medical Publishers, 1975; 75
9. Kasper W., Meinertz T., Henkel B., Eissner D ., Hahn K., Hofmann T., Zeiher A., Just H.:

Echocardiographic findings in patients with proved pulmonary embolism. Am. Heart J. 1986; 112: 1284

10. Fridl P., Jandova R., Stanek V., Fabian J.: The use of suprasternal echocardiography in assessment of pulmonary hypertension (abstr). Washington, X World Congr. Cardiol. 1986; Abstract Book: 273

11. Tramarin R., Torbicki A., Marchandise B., Laaban J.P., Morpurgo M.: European cooperative study on echo-Doppler evaluation of pulmonary artery pressure in patients with chronic lung disease. Eur. Heart J. 1991; 12: 103

12. Ryan T., Petrovic O., Dillon J.C., Feigenbaum H., Conley M.J., Armstrong W.F.: An echocardiographic index for separation of right ventricular volume and pressure overload. J. Am. Coll. Cardiol. 1985; 5: 918

13. Shimada R., Takeshita A., Nakamura M.: Noninvasive assessment of right ventricular systolic pressure in atrial septal defect: Analysis of the end-systolic configuration of the ventricular septum by two-dimensional echocardiography. Am. J. Cardiol. 1984; 53: 1117

14. Morpurgo M., Saviotti M., Dickele, Casazza F., Torbicki A., Weitzenblum E., Zielinski J.: Echocardiographic aspects of pulmonary hypertension in chronic lung disease. Bull. Eur. Physiopathol. Respir. 1984; 20: 251

15. Tanaka H., Tei C., Nakao S., Tahaza M., Sakurai S., Kashima T., Kanehiso T.: Diastolic bulging of the interventricular septum toward the left ventricle. An echocardiographic manifestation of negative interventricular pressure gradient between left and right ventricle during diastole. Circulation 1980; 62: 558

16. Torbicki A., Hawrylkiewicz I., Zielinski J.: Value of M-mode echocardiography in assessing pulmonary arterial pressure in patients with chronic lung disease. Bull. Eur. Physiopathol. Respir. 1987; 23: 233

17. Hirschfelt S., Meyer R., Schwartz D.C., Korfhagen J., Kaplan S.: The echocardiographic assessment of pulmonary artery pressure and pulmonary vascular resistance. Circulation 1975; 52: 642

18. Grose R., Strain J., Ypintosol T.: Right ventricular function in valvular heart disease. Relation to pulmonary artery pressure. J. Am. Coll. Cardiol. 1983; 2: 225

19. Hsieh K.S., Sanders S.P., Colan S.D., MacPherson D., Holland C.: Right ventricular systolic time intervals: Comparison of echocardiographic and Doppler-derived values. Am. Heart J. 1986; 112: 103

20. Torbicki A., Skwarski K., Hawrylkiewicz I., Pasierski T., Miskiewicz Z., Zielinski J.: Comparison of three Doppler methods in the prediction of PAP in patients with chronic lung disease. Eur. Respir. J. 1989; 2: 856

21. Boyd M.J., Williams I.P., Turton C.W.G., Brooks N., Leech G., Millard F.J.C.: Echocardiographic method for the estimation of pulmonary artery pressure in chronic lung disease. Thorax 1980; 85: 914

22. Staring M.R., Crawford M.H., Sorensen S.G., O'Rourke R.A.: A new two-dimensional echocardiographic technique for evaluating right ventricular size and performance in patients with obstructive lung disease. Circulation 1982; 66: 612

23. Weyman A.E., Dillon J.G., Feigenbaum H., Chang S.: Echocardiographic patterns of pulmonary valve motion with pulmonary hypertension. Circulation 1974; 50: 905

24. Zeiher A.M., Bonzel T., Wollschläger H., Hohnloser S., Huse M.H., Just H.: Noninvasive evaluation of pulmonary hypertension by quantitative contrast M-mode echocardiography. Am. Heart J. 1986; 11: 297

25. Kitabatake A., Inoue M., Asao M., Masuyama T., Tanouchi J., Morita T., Mishima M., Uematsu M., Shimazu T., Hori M., Abe H.: Non-invasive evaluation of pulmonary hypertension by a pulsed wave Doppler technique. Circulation 1983; 68: 302

26. Bauman W., Wann L.S., Childress R., Weyman A.E., Dillon J.: Midsystolic notching of the pulmonary valve in the absence of pulmonary hypertension. Am. J. Cardiol. 1979; 43: 1049

90

27. Turkevich D., Groves B.M., Micco A., Trapp J.A.: Early partial systolic closure of the pulmonic valve relates to severity of pulmonary hypertension. Am. Heart J. 1988; 115: 409

28. Marchandise B., De Bruyne B., Delaunois L., Kremer R.: Noninvasive prediction of pulmonary hypertension in chronic obstructive pulmonary disease by Doppler echocardiography. Chest 1987; 91: 361

29. Tramarin R., Colombo E., Opasich C., Fracchia C., Cobelli F.: Subcostal approach in pulsed Doppler evaluation of pulmonary arterial pressure in patients with chronic obstructive pulmonary disease (abstr). Atemw.-Lungenkrkh. 1987; 13: 135

30. Dabestani A., Mahan G., Gardin J., Takenaka K., Burn C., Allfie A., Henry W.L.: Evaluation of pulmonary artery pressure and resistance by pulsed Doppler echocardiography. Am. J. Cardiol. 1987; 59: 662

31. Graettinger W.F., Greene E.R., Voyles W.F.: Doppler predictions of pulmonary artery pressure, flow, and resistance in adults. Am. Heart J. 1987; 113: 1426

32. Isobe M., Yazaki Y., Takaku F., Koizumi K., Hara K., Tsuneyoshi H., Yamaguchi T., Machii K.: Prediction of pulmonary arterial pressure in adults by pulsed Doppler echocardiography. Am. J. Cardiol. 1986; 57: 316

33. Kosturakis D., Goldberg S.J., Allen H.D., Loeber C.: Doppler echocardiographic prediction of pulmonary arterial hypertension in congenital heart disease. Am. J. Cardiol. 1984; 53: 1110

34. Martin-Duran R., Larman M., Trugeda A., De Prada V., Ruano J., Torres A., Figueroa A., Pajaron A., Nistal F.: Comparison of Doppler-determined elevated pulmonary arterial pressure measured at cardiac catheterization. Am. J. Cardiol. 1986; 57: 859

35. Robinson P.J., Macartney F.J., Wyse R.K.H.: Non-invasive diagnosis of pulmonary hypertension. Intern. J. Cardiol. 1986; 11: 253

36. Okamoto M., Miyatake K., Kinoshita N., Sakakibara H., Nimura Y.: Analysis of blood flow in pulmonary hypertension with the pulsed Doppler flowmeter combined with cross sectional echocardiography. Br. Heart J. 1984; 51: 407

37. Panidis I.P., Ross J., Mintz G.S.: Effect of sampling site on assessment of pulmonary artery blood flow by Doppler echocardiography. Am. J. Cardiol. 1986; 58: 1145

38. Matsuda M., Sekiguchi T., Sugishita Y., Kuwako K., Iida K., Ito I.: Reliability of non-invasive estimates of pulmonary hypertension by pulsed Doppler echocardiography. Br. Heart J. 1986; 56: 158

39. Vaska K., Sagar K., Wann L.S.: Pulmonary Doppler ultrasound depends on right ventricular inotropic state as well as pulmonary artery systolic pressure (abstr.). Circulation, 1988; (Suppl. II) 78: 402

40. Cooper M.J., Tyndall M., Silverman N.H.: Evaluation of the responsiveness of elevated pulmonary vascular resistance in children by Doppler echocardiography. J. Am. Coll. Cardiol. 1988; 12: 470

41. Nanna M., Shoalin L., McKay C., Trigleth M., Choudry S., Rahimtoola S.H., Chandraratna P.: Inaccuracy of pulsed Doppler technique in estimating mean pulmonary artery and pulmonary wedge pressure in an unselected population (abstr). J. Am. Coll. Cardiol. 1986; 7: 30A

42. Nanda N.C., Gramiak R., Robinson T.I., Shah P.M.: Echocardiographic evaluation of pulmonary hypertension. Circulation 1974; 50: 575

43. Green S.E., Popp R.L.: The relationship of pulmonary valve motion to the motion of surrounding cardiac structures: a twodimensional and dual M-mode echocardiographic study. Circulation 1981; 64: 107

44. Pocoski D.J., Shah P.M.: Physiologic correlations of pulmonary valve motion in diastole. Circulation 1978; 58: 1064

45. Burstin L.: Determination of pressure in the pulmonary artery by external graphic recordings. Br. Heart J. 1967; 29: 396

46. Hatle L., Angelsen B.A.J., Tromsdal A.: Non-invasive estimation of pulmonary artery systolic pressure with Doppler ultrasound. Br. Heart J. 1981; 45: 157

47. Stevenson J.G., Kawabori I., Guntheroth W.G.: Noninvasive estimation of peak pulmonary artery pressure by M-mode echocardiography. J. Am. Coll. Cardiol. 1984; 4: 1021

48. Burstin L.: The influence of heart rate on isovolumic relaxation. Br. Heart J., 1973; 35: 396

49. Chan K.L., Currie P.J., Seward J.B., Hagler D.J., Mair D.D., Tajik A.J.: Comparison of three Doppler ultrasound methods in the prediction of pulmonary artery pressure. J. Am. Coll. Cardiol. 1987; 9: 549

50. Currie P.J., Seward J.B., Chan K.L., Fyfe D.A., Hagler D.J., Mair D.D., Reeder G.S., Nishimura R.A., Tajik J.A.: Continuous wave Doppler determination of right ventricular pressure: A simultaneous Doppler-catheterization study in 127 patients. J. Am. Coll. Cardiol. 1985; 6: 750

51. Berger M., Haimowitz A., Van Tosh A., Berdoff R.L., Golderg E.: Quantitative assessment of pulmonary hypertension in patients with tricuspid regurgitation using continuous wave Doppler ultrasound. J. Am. Coll. Cardiol. 1985; 6: 359

52. Skjaerpe T., Hatle L.: Noninvasive estimation of systolic pressure in the right ventricle in patients with tricuspid regurgitation. Eur. Heart J. 1986; 7: 704

53. Nakao S., Come P.C., McKay R., Ransil B.J.: Effects of positional changes on inferior vena caval size and dynamics and correlations with right-sided pressure. Am. J. Cardiol. 1987; 59: 125

54. Simonson J.S., Schiller N.B.: Sonospirometry: A new method for noninvasive estimation of mean right atrial pressure based on two-dimensional echographic measurements of the inferior vena cava during measured inspiration. J. Am. Coll. Cardiol. 1988; 11: 557

55. Laaban J.P., Diebold B., Raffoul H., Lafay M., Poirier T., Rochemaure J., Peronneau M.: Noninvasive estimation of systolic pulmonary artery pressure using continuous wave Doppler ultrasound in COPD (abstr.). Am. Rev. Respir. Dis. 1988; 137: 150

56. Beard J.T., Byrd B.F.: Saline contrast enhancement of trivial Doppler tricuspid regurgitation signals for estimating pulmonary artery pressure. Am. J. Cardiol. 1988; 62: 486

57. Himelman R.B., Stulbarg M., Kircher B., Lae E., Kee L., Dean N.C., Golden J., Wolfe C.L., Schiller N.B.: Noninvasive evaluation of pulmonary pressure during exercise by saline-enhanced Doppler echocardiography in chronic pulmonary disease. Circulation 1975; 52: 642

58. Marx G.R., Allen H.D., Goldberg S.J.: Doppler echocardiographic estimation of systolic pulmonary artery pressure in pediatric patients with interventricular communications. J. Am. Coll. Cardiol. 1985; 6: 1133

59. Matsuoka Y., Hayakawa K.: Noninvasive estimation of right ventricular systolic pressure in ventricular septal defect by a continuous wave Doppler technique. Jpn. Circ. J. 1986; 50: 1062

60. Michelsen S., Hurlen M., Otterstad J.E.: Prevalence of tricuspid and pulmonary regurgitation diagnosed by Doppler in apparently healthy women. Possible influence on their physical performance? Eur. Heart J. 1988; 9: 61

61. Yock P.G., Popp R.L.: Noninvasive estimation of right ventricular systolic pressure by Doppler ultrasound in patients with tricuspid regurgitation. Circulation 1984; 70: 657

62. Takao S., Miyatake K., Izumi S., Okamoto M., Kinoshita N., Nakagawa H., Yamamoto K., Sakakibara H., Nimura Y.: Clincal implications of pulmonary regurgitation in healthy individuals: Detection by cross sectional pulsed Doppler echocardiography. Br. Heart J. 1988; 59: 542

63. Masuyama T., Kcdama K., Kitabatake A., Sato H., Nanto S., Inoue M.: Continuous wave Doppler echocardiographic detection of pulmonary regurgitation and its application to noninvasive estimation of pulmonary artery pressure. Circulation 1986; 74: 484

Respiratory Failure

10. Ventilatory Failure

L. Appendini,[1] A. Rossi[2]

1. Division of Pulmonary Disease, Clinica del Lavoro Foundation, Institute of Care and
   Research, Medical Center of Rehabilitation, Veruno, Italy
2. Respiratory Division, O.C.M., U.S.L. 25, Verona, and Department of Internal
   Medicine, University of Verona, Italy

Introduction

The goal of respiration is to bring oxygen to tissues and to take carbon dioxide away from tissues. The respiratory and cardiocirculatory systems cooperate in this task. The former deals with the transfer of respiratory gases (oxygen and carbon dioxide) between air and blood, whereas the latter brings respiratory gases from blood to tissues and vice versa. To achieve these goals, both systems are composed of a gas exchanger (the lungs and the capillary bed, respectively) and of a mechanical pump (the respiratory muscles and the heart). Therefore respiratory failure can be due to gas exchanger and/or to pump failure in both respiratory and cardiocirculatory systems. We will focus our attention on the failure of the respiratory system, particularly on pump failure.

As mentioned above, the respiratory system is composed of two parts, a gas exchanger (the lungs) in which oxygen passes from alveoli to blood and carbon dioxide from blood to alveoli, and a pump which acts on the lungs to bring fresh air into and alveolar gases out of the gas exchanger.[1]

Lung Failure

Failure of gas exchange in the lungs is the result of ventilation/perfusion ($\dot{V}A/\dot{Q}$) imbalance, intrapulmonary shunts, or impairment of diffusion equilibrium across alveolar capillary membrane. These mechanisms can currently cause hypoxemia but not hypercapnia. Ventilation/perfusion mismatching contributes to hypoxemia by means of two mechanisms. The first involves the sigmoid shape of the Hb-O$_2$ dissociation curve, so that the blood perfusing the high $\dot{V}A/\dot{Q}$ alveoli will have little extra O$_2$ content, while the blood perfusing the low $\dot{V}A/\dot{Q}$ alveoli will have significantly less O$_2$ content than normal. Then, the mixed pulmonary venous blood O$_2$ content, and hence PaO$_2$, will be significantly reduced.

The second mechanism acts through differences between regional blood flow that, even in normal subjects, are greater in the low $\dot{V}A/\dot{Q}$ regions.[2] On the other hand, since the CO$_2$ dissociation curve is so much steeper than is the Hb-O$_2$ dissociation curve, PaCO$_2$ is less affected by ventilation/perfusion mismatching. In other words, the low CO$_2$ content of high $\dot{V}A/\dot{Q}$ alveoli tends to cancel out the high CO$_2$ content of low $\dot{V}A/\dot{Q}$ alveoli. Furthermore, moderately large changes in CO$_2$ content of blood can occur without changing the PaCO$_2$ by more than a few millimeters of mercury. Intrapulmonary shunt can be considered as an extreme case of ventilation/perfusion mismatching in which the ratio is equal to 0. In this case, the mechanisms that produce hypoxemia are the same, but this last can not be corrected by increasing the oxygen inspiratory fractional content (FIO$_2$). This factor must be taken into account in patients with status asthmaticus requiring mechanical ventilation in which a considerable increase in shunt when given 100% O$_2$ was recently demonstrated.[3] On the other hand, administration of 100% O$_2$ does not increase pulmonary shunting in chronic obstructive pulmonary disease (COPD) either during mechanical ventilation, or during spontaneous ventilation after weaning, although in this latter the dispersion of the pulmonary blood flow distribution increases, suggesting release of hypoxic pulmonary vasoconstriction.[4]

Gas transfer across alveolar capillary membrane can be diffusion-limited or perfusion-limited. Usually, in normal subjects, both oxygen and carbon dioxide transfer are only perfusion-limited. Nevertheless, fibrotic thickening of alveolar membranes or interstitial edema may be responsible for the diffusion limitation of the oxygen transfer during strenuous exercise, whereas only extremely abnormal alveolar-capillary barrier might be the cause of diffusion limitation of oxygen transfer even at rest.[5] On the other hand, carbon dioxide generally achieves equilibration between alveolar gas and blood, because of its much greater diffusibility (i.e. it diffuses about 20 times as easily as O$_2$ does).

Pump Failure

Failure of the pump leads mainly to alveolar hypoventilation, which in turn is responsible for hypercapnia.[1] In normal subjects, and to some extent in many patients with a variety of respiratory diseases, PaCO$_2$ and pH remain constant even if the respiratory system has to face significant changes of the metabolic rate. At rest, PaCO$_2$ is less than 45 millimeters of mercury independently of age (up to 80 years old), and of body position. In some patients, however, the ventilatory pump can be altered to the extent that, at rest and breathing room air, adequate alveolar ventilation can not be maintained and hypercapnia develops. The relationship between $PaCO_2$ and alveolar ventilation is described by the following respiratory equation:

$$PaCO_2 = \dot{V}CO_2 \times K/\dot{V}A = \dot{V}CO_2 \times K/\dot{V}E(1-Vd/VT) \qquad (1)$$

where $\dot{V}CO_2 = CO_2$ metabolic production; K = constant; $\dot{V}A$ = alveolar ventilation; $\dot{V}E$ = minute ventilation; VT = tidal volume; Vd = physiologic dead space. At any given level of $\dot{V}CO_2$, a decrease of $\dot{V}A$ results in an increase of $PaCO_2$ and vice versa.

Equation (1) also shows that $PaCO_2$ depends on the pattern of breathing. For example, at constant $\dot{V}E$ and Vd, $\dot{V}A$ is reduced as VT decreases and breathing frequency (f) increases. Moreover, VT can be affected by the rate of increase of pulmonary volume (VT/TI), by the duration of the inspiratory cycle (TI), or by both these factors. Furthermore, breathing frequency f can be modified by changes of TI or TE or by both. Finally, it has been suggested that VT/TI, TI and TE are independently controlled by different nervous pathways such as vagal and non-vagal reflexes, or by chemoreceptor stimulation.[6]

The interaction between these mechanisms determines the ventilatory cycle. Even if the "weight" of each mechanism is not known, ventilatory cycle (and then minute ventilation) can be usefully divided in a "driving" and a "timing" component as follows:[7]

$$\dot{V}E = (VT/TI) \times (TI/TTOT) \qquad (2)$$

where the mean inspiratory flow VT/TI represents an index of the driving neural mechanism, and $TI/TTOT$ depends on the timing control mechanism.

The mean inspiratory flow represents the mechanical output of the ventilatory pump according to the following sequence:

1. the respiratory centers stimulate respiratory muscles through neural efferent pathways and motoneurons;
2. respiratory muscles shorten and displace the chest wall and the lungs to produce the driving intrathoracic and alveolar pressure that generates flow;
3. afferent nervous pathways modulate respiratory centers output to muscles.

Any impairment in this chain of events leads to a reduction of the mechanical output of the pump, and then to hypercapnia.

Inadequate Central Respiratory Drive

Traditionally, control of breathing has been assessed by means of ventilatory response to CO_2, hypoxemia, and exercise. These methods seem to be effective when the impairment lies inside the respiratory control system itself, as congenital neurological disorders (i.e. Ondine syndrome), drug overdose, or pharmacological depression. But, as mentioned above, ventilatory response reflects not only how much a patient "wants to breathe", but also how much the failure of the other components of the pump "allows him to breathe" or how much "he can breathe". A significant effort has been devoted to investigating the role of motor neuron discharge failure,[8] neuromuscular coupling,[9] contractility of respiratory muscles,[10] abnormal chest wall and lung mechanics[11,12] in the reduction of mechanical output of the respiratory pump in spite of adequate neural drive.

The techniques used in several studies, i.e. electroneurography, electromyography of the diaphragm, the measurement of transdiaphragmatic pressure, the work of breathing, and the oxygen cost of ventilation are somewhat complex, sophisticated, and sometimes invasive. More flexible, even if not faultless, is the measurement of the mouth occlusion pressure (P0.1) as index of respiratory center output. Briefly, it consists in the measurement of the pressure generated at the mouth 100 milliseconds after the beginning of an inspiratory effort from the relaxation volume (Vr) against the occluded airway.[13] P0.1 represents the net airway pressure available to produce inspiratory flow that is generated by the neurochemical drive present at the beginning of inspiration. It has the advantage of being non-invasive and relatively unaffected by respiratory mechanics.[13] However, like other measurements P0.1 has some limitations because it is not a direct estimate of the inspiratory neural drive. Indeed, the transduction of the electrical signal (nervous signal) into a mechanical output (pressure at the mouth) is mediated by such factors as pulmonary volume, mechanical coupling, activation of muscles other than inspiratory muscles, airways compliance, etc. An exhaustive review of these factors has been previously done.[6] In spite of these limits, P0.1 represents a useful clinical index in the assessment of respiratory drive.

Inspiratory Muscle Fatigue

There is ample evidence that, in patients with high airways resistance or with low respiratory system compliance, respiratory drive (i.e. P0.1) is high, and that ventilatory failure depends on the inefficiency in the conversion of neural drive into airflow.[6] This view was formalized in 1982 by Roussos et al. in a classic representation in which ventilatory pump failure, in absence of respiratory centers impairment, was ascribed to a mechanical defect of the pump or to respiratory muscle fatigue.[1]

In general, this latter was defined as the inability of a muscle to continue to generate a required force as the result of an imbalance between its energy supply and demand.[1] In the respiratory system, it was considered as the inability to continue to generate the pressure required to maintain an adequate alveolar ventilation.[1] Fatigue would ensue from reduced energy supply in cardiogenic shock,[14] from strenuous inspiratory muscle contraction that limits their blood flow,[15] and from poor nutritional status, catabolic states or prolonged submaximal breathing in which energy stores could be depleted.[16]

Furthermore, inspiratory muscle fatigue could also be the result of increased demands when airways resistance is high and efficiency of contraction is decreased as in asthma or chronic airflow limitation, or when respiratory system compliance is reduced as in interstitial lung disease or fibrothorax.[1] In addition, since hypercapnia can be of acute or chronic onset, it was postulated that inspiratory muscle fatigue could also be acute and chronic.[1]

More recently, muscle fatigue has been re-defined as follows:[17] "muscle fatigue is a condition in which there is a loss in the capacity for developing force and/or velocity of a muscle, resulting from muscle activity under load and which is reversible by rest".This new definition points out some crucial aspects.

1. Muscle fatigue is defined by muscle force loss and not by task failure. This implies that inspiratory muscle fatigue cannot be identified with acute or chronic ventilatory failure, whereas it can precede the function impairment. The evidence that electromyogram pattern of inspiratory muscle fatigue appears before that of mechanical failure[18] supports the previous statement. Hence, it is possible that changes in electromyogram power spectrum of inspiratory muscles accurately track the time course of fatigue onset.[19]
2. The load on muscles is recognized as the causal factor acting against muscles to determine their fatigue. The importance of inspiratory muscle loading is stressed by the evidence that such a clinical sign as paradoxical motion of the abdominal wall, considered a manifestation of inspiratory muscle fatigue,[20] was demonstrated to be present during respiratory loading in absence of signs of inspiratory muscle fatigue.[21]
3. The occurrence of recovery of force and/or velocity loss with rest allows the distinction between "fatigue" and "weakness" of inspiration muscles. According to the above definition, weakness is a muscle condition that can not take advantage of rest.[17,19] Clinical examples are myasthenia gravis and amyotrophic lateral sclerosis. This distinction has important therapeutic consequences. First, in presence of ventilatory failure consequent to inspiratory muscle fatigue, ventilatory muscle rest (VMR) could reverse both conditions. Controversial clinical results on VMR have been reported.[22] The uncertainty about the diagnosis of inspiratory muscle fatigue can explain these contrasting results. Second, putting into rest inspiratory muscles that are not fatigued could lead to their atrophy.[1] Third, if chronic fatigue exists, it is unlikely that a chronically fatigued muscle could be trained.[12] On the contrary, the evidence of muscle weakness strongly supports the use of inspiratory muscle training (IMT).

Clinical results were obtained pro and con also in this field.[22,23] Apart from methodological problems that can affect these results,[23] the baseline status of inspiratory muscles should be taken in account to explain the different outcomes of training. The conclusion that can be drawn is that a punctual assessment of inspiratory muscle status is mandatory to treat successfully at least chronic ventilatory failure by means of VMR or IMT.

Whatever the role played by inspiratory muscle fatigue or weakness in ventilatory failure, it clearly appears to be determined by an imbalance between inspiratory muscle contraction and the load applied.

Inspiratory Muscle Load

The load on inspiratory muscles is elastic and resistive in nature. Elastic load is typically increased in restrictive pulmonary disease.[24] On the other hand, early studies suggested that the compliance of the respiratory system may be increased in COPD. However, Sharp et al. found that under anesthesia and neuromuscular paralysis the pressure volume (PV) relation is simply shifted upward, the slope of the relation near passive FRC being similar to normals.[25]

This study demonstrated that, if COPD patients breathed near their passive FRC, their elastic load would be normal and it would not compromise the conversion of neuromuscular drive into ventilation. If in COPD patients static compliance results are normal, the dynamic compliance of the respiratory system can, however, be reduced for at least two reasons. First, the frequency dependence of dynamic compliance is greatly increased.[26] Second, dynamic factors such as the post-inspiratory activity of inspiratory muscles or the increased airflow resistance and breathing frequency can raise the end expiratory lung volume (EELV) above the relaxation volume of the respiratory system.[27]

These two latter mechanisms determine the presence of a positive elastic recoil pressure at end expiration (intrinsic positive end expiratory pressure, PEEPi), ranging from a few centimeters of water in stable COPD patients[28,29] to as high as 22 cmH$_2$O during acute respiratory failure.[30] The higher EELV shifts tidal volume in a stiffer range of the PV curve,[31] increasing the elastic work performed by inspiratory muscles. In addition, inspiratory muscles have also to generate an extra pressure to counterbalance PEEPi before inspiratory flow can begin.[32]

In absence of expiratory flow limitation, inspiratory and expiratory increase of flow resistance can be faced by respiratory muscles with minor adjustments in respiratory output.[31]

On the other hand, the reduction in expiratory $\dot{V}$max is the main determinant of expiratory time prolongation. Indeed, in presence of expiratory flow limitation, the time needed for a complete exhalation to Vr is longer than the expiratory time set by respiratory centers. This imbalance leads to incomplete emptying of tidal volume (dynamic hyperinflation, DH) and, as consequence, to PEEPi onset.[28]

Dynamic hyperinflation is crucial to challenge inspiratory muscle function. Apart from the threshold load represented by PEEPi, hyperinflation can decrease the pressure developed by inspiratory muscles since they become shifted from their optimal length of contraction.[1]

This could be not true when hyperinflation is chronic (i.e. in the case of increased lung compliance), since plastic remodeling within the inspiratory muscles can result in a new "optimal" operating length[33] with loss of sarcomeres.[34]

Very different is the situation in which hyperinflation has an acute onset, as occurs during acute respiratory failure (ARF). In this case DH can be more than 1.3 liters above Vr[30] and the relative shift of muscle fibers from their optimal length of contraction can not be compensated for, resulting in a great impairment of the muscles, ability to generate pressure. Furthermore, there is the evidence that, with increasing lung volume, the diaphragm becomes less effective in inflating the rib cage.[1] The diaphragm promotes inspiration through the appositional and insertional components of its contraction on the rib cage.

With increasing lung volume, the area of apposition decreases, and therefore the expiratory action through pleural pressure increases. Finally, at very high lung volumes, the zone of apposition completely disappears, the diaphragmatic fibers are directed centrally rather than in a cephalic direction, and the contraction of the diaphragm under these conditions tends to pull inward the lower rib cage, causing less negative intrapleural pressure and a direct expiratory effect.

In summary, in absence of dynamic hyperinflation, elastic and resistive loading could have modest effects on neuro-ventilatory coupling. On the other hand, dynamic hyperinflation greatly impairs the pressure-generating characteristics of inspiratory muscles, whereas a threshold load is added to an increased elastic load.

Since PEEPi and dynamic hyperinflation play a paramount role in inspiratory muscle function impairment and in ventilatory failure onset, attempts have been made to treat it by means of external continuous positive airway pressure (CPAP). This topic has been recently reviewed.[35] It is then possible to postulate that ventilatory failure of acute onset would be prevented by de-loading inspiratory muscles in these patients.

Ventilation-Stimulation Coupling

Afferent signals arising from the ventilatory pump to the respiratory centers can have an important influence on central respiratory drive and can be a determinant factor of ventilatory failure.[36] There is recent evidence that hypercapnia occurs when the inspiratory muscles are required to develop a tidal pressure greater than one-third of maximal inspiratory pressure.[37]

Furthermore it is well documented that, when hypercapnic patients are asked to reduce their $PaCO_2$ by increasing their VT, inspiratory muscle fatigue ensues.[38] These data suggest that inspiratory muscle loading may modulate the central ventilatory drive to prevent inspiratory muscle fatigue and failure.[37] The pathway of this reflex activity seems to travel via phrenic afferents,[39] and to act on the timing component of the ventilatory cycle with a reduction of Ti.

If tachipnea is the natural response to the combination of elastic load and weakness of the inspiratory muscles,[40] it seems surprising that flow limitation could be associated with this pattern of breathing,[41] since normal subjects' response to inspiratory and expiratory resistive load is a reduced breathing frequency and an increased tidal volume.[42,43] A possible explanation lies in that the prevalent load on inspiratory muscles is dynamic hyperinflation that, as stated above, leads to a combination of elastic load and inspiratory threshold load coupled with inspiratory muscle weakness. Then, the slowing effect on breathing frequency expected in response to high inspiratory and expiratory resistance[44] would be contrasted by the stronger tachipneic effect of elastic loading and inspiratory muscle weakness.[40] Unfortunately, this latter response, that is set to minimize the mean inspiratory pressure required to produce a given ventilation and, in consequence, to de-load inspiratory muscles, paradoxically damages them. In fact, the increase of breathing frequency causes further hyperinflation and, so doing, it further increases the threshold and elastic loads in a closed loop. Finally, the increase of breathing frequency and the shortening of Ti lead to hypercapnia as discussed above (see Pump Failure).

In conclusion, ventilatory failure can result from the impairment of each component of the ventilatory pump or from the interaction between an injured component and the rest of the ventilatory machinery. Furthermore, gas exchange failure in the lungs and ventilatory failure in the pump can coexist and interact. A better comprehension of these mechanisms is mandatory to add new knowledge on ventilatory failure and to improve its treatment.

References

1. Roussos C., Macklem P.T.: The respiratory muscles: medical progress. N. Engl. J. Med. 1982; 307: 786-797
2. West J.B.: Ventilation/blood flow and gas exchange. 3rd ed, Oxford, Blackwell, 1977; 33-52
3. Rodriguez-Roisin R., Ballester E., Roca J., Torres A., Wagner P.D.: Mechanisms of hypoxemia in patients with status asthmaticus requiring mechanical ventilation. Am. Rev. Respir. Dis. 1989; 139: 732-739
4. Torres A., Reyes A., Roca J., Wagner P.D., Rodriguez-Roisin R.: Ventilation-perfusion mismatching in chronic obstructive pulmonary disease during ventilator weaning. Am. Rev. Respir. Dis. 1989; 140: 1246-1250
5. Wagner P.D., West J.B.: Effects of diffusion impairment on O_2 and CO_2 time courses in

pulmonary capillaries. J. Appl. Physiol. 1972; 33: 62-71

6. Milic-Emili J.: Recent advances in clinical assessment of control of breathing. Lung 1982; 160: 1-17

7. Milic-Emili J., Grunstein M.M.: Drive and timing components of ventilation. Chest 1976; 70(suppl): 131-133

8. Valli G., Barbieri S., Sergi P., Fayoumi Z., Berardinelli P.: Evidence of motor neuron involvement in chronic respiratory insufficiency. J. Neurol. Neurosurg. Psychiatry 1984; 47: 1117-1121

9. Haxhiu M.A., Cherniack N.S., Altose M.D., Kelsen S.G.: Effect of respiratory loading on the relationship between occlusion pressure and diaphragm EMG during hypoxia and hypercapnia. Am. Rev. Respir. Dis. 1983; 127: 185-188

10. Moxham J., Wiles C.M., Newham D., Edwards R.H.T.: Contractile function and fatigue of the respiratory muscles in man. In: *Human Muscle Fatigue: Physiological Mechanisms*. Pitman Medical 1982, London: 197-212. (Ciba Foundation Symposium '82).

11. Marazzini L., Cavestri R., Gori D., Gatti L., Longhini E.: Difference between mouth and esophageal occlusion pressure during CO_2 rebreathing in chronic obstructive pulmonary disease. Am. Rev. Respir. Dis. 1978; 118: 1027-1033

12. Macklem P.T.: Hyperinflation. Am. Rev. Respir. Dis. 1984; 129: 1-2

13. Whitelaw W.A., Derenne J.P., Milic-Emili J.: Occlusion pressure as a measure of respiratory center output in conscious man. Respir. Physiol. 1975; 23: 181-199

14. Aubier M., Trippenbach T., Roussos C.H.: Respiratory muscles fatigue during cardiogenic shock. J. Appl. Physiol. 1981; 51: 499-508

15. Bellemare F., Wight D., Lavigne C.M., Grassino A.: Limitation of diaphragmatic blood flow in dogs. Fed. Proc. 1982; 41: 1255 (abstract).

16. Gertz J., Hedenstierna G., Hellers G., Wahren J.: Muscle metabolism in patients with chronic obstructive lung disease and acute respiratory failure. Clin. Sci. Mol. Med. 1977; 52: 395-403

17. NHLBI Workshop: Respiratory muscle fatigue. Report of the respiratory muscle fatigue workshop group. Am. Rev. Respir. Dis. 1990; 142: 474-480

18. Grassino A., Macklem P.T.: Respiratory muscle fatigue and ventilatory failure. Am. Rev. Med. 1984; 35: 625-647

19. Macklem P.T.: The importance of defining respiratory muscle fatigue. Am. Rev. Respir. Dis. 1990; 142: 274

20. Cohen C., Zagelbaum G., Gross D., Roussos C., Macklem P.T.: Clinical manifestations of inspiratory muscle fatigue. Am. J. Med. 1982; 73: 308-316

21. Tobin M.J., Perez W., Guenther S.M., Lodato R.F., Dantzker D.R: Does rib cage-abdominal paradox signify respiratory muscle fatigue? J. Appl. Physiol. 1987; 63(2): 851-860

22. Martin J.G.: Clinical intervention in chronic respiratory failure. Chest 1990; 97(3): 105S-109S

23. Grassino A: Inspiratory muscle training in COPD patients. Eur. Respir. J. 1989; 2 (suppl 7): 581S-586S

24. Renzi G., Milic-Emili J., Grassino A.: Control of breathing in diffuse lung fibrosis. Bull. Eur. Physiopathol. Respir. 1981; 18: 461-472

25. Sharp J.T., Lith P.V., Nuchprayoon C.V., Brinev R., Johnson F.N.: The thorax in chronic obstructive lung disease. Am. J. Med. 1968; 44: 39-46

26. Pride N.B., Macklem P.T.: Lung mechanics in disease: in: *Handbook of physiology*, vol. 3. *The respiratory system*. Bethesda: Am. Physiolog. Soc., 1986: 659-692

27. Martin J.G., De Troyer A.: The thorax and the control of the functional residual capacity. In: Roussos C and Macklem PT(eds.) *The thorax* (part B). Marcel Dekker Inc, New York, Basel, 1985; 29: 1373-1405

28. Dal Vecchio L., Polese G., Poggi R., Rossi A.: "Intrinsic" positive end-expiratory pressure in

stable patients with chronic obstructive pulmonary disease. Eur. Respir. J. 1990; 3(1): 74-80

29. Haluszka J., Chartrand D.A., Grassino A.E., Milic-Emili J.: Intrinsic PEEP and arterial PCO_2 in stable patients with chronic obstructive pulmonary disease. Am. Rev. Respir. Dis. 1990; 141: 1194-1197

30. Broseghini C., Brandolese R., Poggi R., Polese G., Manzin E., Milic-Emili J., Rossi A.: Respiratory mechanics during the first day of mechanical ventilation in patients with pulmonary edema and chronic airway obstruction. Am. Rev. Respir. Dis. 1988; 138: 355-361

31. Younes M.: Load responses, dyspnea, and respiratory failure. Chest 1990; 97(3): 595-685

32. Milic-Emili J., Gottfried S.B., Rossi A.: Dynamic hyperinflation: intrinsic PEEP and its ramifications in patients with respiratory failure. In: JL Vincent (ed.) Int. Care Med. 1987; 192-198

33. Farkas G.A., Roussos C.: Adaptability of the hamster diaphragm to exercise and/or emphysema. J. Appl. Physiol. 1982; 53: 1263-1272

34. Keens T.G., Bryan A.C., Levison H., Iannuzzo C.D.: Developmental pattern of muscle fiber types in human ventilatory muscles. J. Appl. Physiol. 1978; 44: 909-913

35. Rossi A., Brandolese R., Milic-Emili J., Gottfried S.B.: The role of PEEP in patients with chronic obstructive pulmonary disease during assisted ventilation. Eur. Respir. J. 1990; 3(7): 818-822

36. Ward M., Macklem P.T.: The act of breathing and how it fails. Chest 1990; 97(3): 365-395

37. Begin P, Grassino A: Role of inspiratory muscle function in chronic hypercapnia. Chest 1990; 97(3): 585

38. Grassino A., Bellemare F., Laporta D.: Diaphragm fatigue and the strategy of breathing in COPD. Chest 1984; 855: 51S-54S

39. Yammes Y., Buchler B., Delpierre S., Rasidakis R., Grimand C., Roussos C.: Phrenic afferents and their role in inspiratory control. J. Appl. Physiol. 1986; 60: 854-860

40. Milic-Emili J., Zin W.A.: Breathing responses to imposed mechanical loads. In: *Handbook of physiology, vol. II. The respiratory system.* Bethesda: Am. Physiolog. Soc., 1986: 751-770

41. O' Donnell D.E., Sanii R., Anthonisen N.R., Younes M.: Effect of dynamic airway compression on breathing pattern and respiratory sensation in severe chronic obstructive pulmonary disease. Am. Rev. Respir. Dis. 1987; 135: 912-918

42. Imhof V., West P., Younes M.: Steady state response of normal subjects to inspiratory resistive loads. J. Appl. Physiol. 1986; 60: 1471-1481

43. Poon C.S., Younes M., Gallagher C.G.: Effects of expiratory resistive load on respiratory motor output in conscious humans. J. Appl. Physiol. 1987; 63: 1837-1845

44. Coleridge H.M., Coleridge J.G.C.: Reflexes evoked from tracheobronchial tree and lungs. In: *Handbook of physiology. The respiratory system. Control of breathing.* Bethesda: Am. Physiolog. Soc., 1986; 395-430

11. Metabolism and Nutrition in Rehabilitation of the Patient with Respiratory Insufficiency

R.D. FERRANTI,[1,2] R. MALFA[1]

1. Gaylord Rehabilitation Hospital, Center for Breathing Disorders, Wallingford, CT, USA
2. Yale University Medical School, Section of Pulmonary Disease, New Haven, USA

Introduction

There has always been an understanding of the importance of proper breathing and eating in health and disease. In the past few decades, the relationships between metabolism and respiratory function, in general, and nutrition and ventilation in particular have been more closely investigated and have acquired growing importance in rehabilitation. Malnutrition, metabolic disorders, electrolyte disturbances and abnormalities of gas exchange can have profound effects on ventilation especially through their effects on the ventilatory muscles. When the diagnosis of a condition which may place the patient at risk of respiratory insufficiency is first made, nutritional and metabolic assessment becomes immediately important.

Changes in body weight and metabolic parameters should be closely followed. Serum albumin has been found to be a good predictor of discharge outcome in hospitalized COPD patients, and it has been related to exercise performance in COPD patients. It also appears to be critical in monitoring the weaning of the patients from assisted ventilation and in their discharge planning.

For the rehabilitation of the respiratory patient, metabolic balance and maintenance of nutrition appear no less important than ventilation itself because the two are inextricably related.

Effects of Malnutrition on the Respiratory System

A classification of different types of malnutrition has been criticized as overly simplistic and impeding the understanding of patients with nutritional depletion.[59]

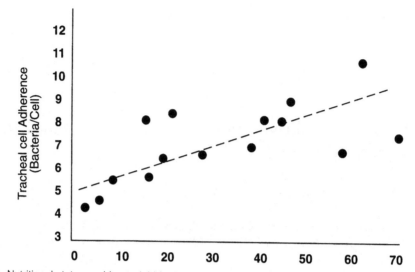

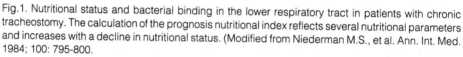

Fig.1. Nutritional status and bacterial binding in the lower respiratory tract in patients with chronic tracheostomy. The calculation of the prognosis nutritional index reflects several nutritional parameters and increases with a decline in nutritional status. (Modified from Niederman M.S., et al. Ann. Int. Med. 1984; 100: 795-800.

However, in general, the term malnutrition is used to mean energy and protein malnutrition or Protein Calorie Malnutrition (PCM). The term Marasmus has also been used to indicate energy or energy plus protein malnutrition. The term Kwashiorkor usually is used to mean protein malnutrition. Selective deficiencies of micronutrients, vitamins and minerals may also occur because of monotonous incomplete dietary habits or iatrogenic intervention.

Malnutrition is associated with hypoventilation,[16,32] reduction of surfactant production,[40,41,50,89] emphysema like changes,[90] altered lung mechanics,[89,45] and consequently the tendency to hypoventilation, atelectasis and failure, especially in patients with ventilatory fatigue or neuromuscular disease.[24,87]

Immunodeficiency has also been described in malnutrition.[29,63,95] Niederman, in a study done in the COPD population at Gaylord Hospital, demonstrated a definite correlation between bacterial adherence to upper airways epithelium and nutritional status, in tracheostomized patients (Fig. 1).[71]

In severe starvation all organ systems which interact in oxygen transport are affected. Severe starvation may result in cardiorespiratory failure and death.[94,106]

Malnutrition and Ventilation

The effect of malnutrition on ventilation can be the result of its impact on the ventilatory muscles. The works of Rochester and his associates focused on the role of the ventilatory muscles, the "respiratory pump". They demonstrated that necropsy studies of the diaphragm of non-obese laborers showed significantly increased mass, thickness, area and length compared to patients who had sedentary occupations and normal weight.[11] In non-COPD, underweight subjects with prolonged illness, diaphragm muscle mass, thickness and area were all significantly reduced proportionate to body weight.[11]

In non-COPD subjects, Body Weight (BW) and muscularity affect diaphragm muscle mass and dimension, showing approximately a threefold variation between normal subjects and underweight patients.[12]

In underweight COPD subjects, while muscle mass was significantly reduced, area and thickness were reduced, but not significantly when compared to normal weight COPD subjects.[10] When normal weight COPD patients were compared to normal weight matched controls, there was no significant difference in diaphragm muscle mass, area and length.[10]

The compensatory diaphragm shortening seen in emphysema induced studies in hamsters[35,97] may not be evident in man until functional residual capacity (FRC) reaches levels two or three times normal, or total lung capacity (TLC) reaches 1.5 times predicted.[10]

Respiratory muscle strength is a primary determinant of maximum voluntary ventilation (MVV) in interstitial lung disease and an important determinant in patients with chronic hyperinflation.[1]

Respiratory muscle strength and maximal voluntary ventilation (MVV) are reduced in malnourished patients.[9]

There is an inverse relationship between Maximal Inspiratory Pressure (Pi max) and arterial partial pressure of Carbon Dioxide ($PaCO_2$): but patients with COPD and hypercapnia ($PaCO_2 > 45$ torr), manifest it at Pimax 50% of predicted, while myopathic patients manifest it at Pi max 30% of predicted. Variances in Pi max are explained better as a combined function of maximal expiratory pressure (Pe max) plus diaphragm length (DLI) than by DLI or Pe max alone or DLI plus BW. These observations suggest that, in COPD patients, in the determination of Pi max, besides the mechanical disadvantage expressed by DLI, there is generalized muscle weakness expressed by Pemax, probably determined by nutritional depletion, plus factors which may be humoral, hormonal or other.[24,85,86]

Other investigators have studied relationships between undernutrition and ventilatory muscle tension.

Studies by Kelsen and associates show that undernutrition decreases the maximum isometric tension generated by the hamster diaphragm at any given muscle length and stimulus frequency. This observation may be explained by reduction in muscle mass rather than in mechanical efficiency, since tension per unit of muscle cross-sectional area or per unit of weight is the same in undernourished and control animals.[57] Lewis and associates observed that in undernourished animals, the rate of fall of isometric tension during repeated stimulation is also affected, and the time required for tension to fall (endurance time) is greater in undernourished than in control animals, although the absolute tension at any point in time is less.

These results are mainly due to reduction in muscle mass and greater atrophy of fast muscle fibers. Slow muscle fibers are more resistant. Atrophy of fast fibers favors fatigue, fatigue being expressed as the level of force generated during breathing as a percentage of the maximum (spontaneously) obtainable force.[65,66]

The Effect of Disease on Respiration

Nutritional needs depend on body size, sex and age, but are also affected by activities and environmental changes and by hormonal, enzymatic and metabolic factors which may be genetic or acquired as result of injury or illness.

The fuel for the human skeletal muscle is carbohydrate and lipid. Blood glucose can be used directly, but it is mostly first converted into glycogen and stored intracellularly. Lipid, in the form of free fatty acid, is the main form of fuel at rest and during low intensity exercise. Lipid metabolism is only aerobic. Carbohydrate can be used aerobically and anaerobically, and it is the fuel of choice for high intensity exercise. As intensity of exercise increases, the need of available carbohydrate also increases.[54]

Inborn errors of muscle metabolism include deficiency of enzymes necessary for lipid metabolism, such as carnitine palmitosyl transferase deficiency,[64] or impairment of carbohydrate assimilation, such as deficiency of muscle phosphoriylase, McArdle syndrome,[77] or of carbohydrate utilization such as in phosphofructokinase deficiency. These diseases, although not common, may affect the ventilatory muscles, and may require special diets and or adequate exercise regimens. In another disorder, acid maltase deficiency, a glycogen storage defect which affects the ventilatory muscles, a diet based on low carbohydrate, high protein and fat reduces ventilator dependency.[31]

In Carnitine deficiency, in contrast, the proper prescription is a high carbohydrate diet and avoidance of prolonged exercise.[64]

Other metabolic, hormonal disorders such as thyroid dysfunction and diabetes are more common in medical practice. The effects of undernutrition and the biochemical and hormonal mechanisms underlying skeletal muscle atrophy have recently been reviewed by Kelsen.[58]

Thyroid hormone in animal studies affects the enzyme activity pattern of the energy-supplying metabolism of muscle fibers.[60] In thyroid dysfunction, both hypo- and hyperthyroidism, ventilation is affected.

Therapeutic regulation of thyroid activity normalizes symptomatology. Hypothyroidism can be a cause for ventilatory dependency, and replacement therapy in these patients often allows for weaning.

Diabetes decreases the activity of glycolytic pathways (Phosphorylase, Hexokinase, Phosphofructokinase) without significant changes of important oxidative enzymes (succinic dehydrogenase and citrate synthase).[53] But it has also been reported to blunt the adaptive changes in oxidative and glycolytic enzyme activity induced in the diaphragm by endurance training,[53] and to accelerate activity of lysozomal protease, and decrease protein synthesis.[42,43,68,75] These effects are greater in fast twitch and mixed fibers than in slow twitch fibers. Insulin replacement reverses the effects of streptozotocin induced diabetes on the diaphragm in animals.[46] Pulmonary functions are decreased in diabetic individuals, in particular VC.[62,79] Diabetes and hyperglycemia are often noted in patients with severe respiratory insufficiency and failure.

We conducted a preliminary retrospective pilot study in forty-three patients who were referred to our rehabilitation unit in one year because of difficulty in weaning from the ventilator or because of recurrent related problems (43 patients, 56 admissions). Serum Albumin (SA), Glucose (G), and Creatinine (C) values were extracted from admission and discharge data, along with ventilatory outcome; either weaned, on nocturnal ventilation or full time ventilation, and discharge outcome; home, acute care, extended care facility, or expired.

Analysis showed that hyperglycemia was the most prevalent abnormality, probably due to the common use of steroids in this population, prevalently COPD. Abnormalities of two or all three parameters were frequent. However only admission SA showed the strongest predicting value for weaning completely or partially from the ventilator and for discharge home (Figs. 2 and 3) G or C did not show significant influence on outcome.

A prior study, at Gaylord Hospital, found SA to be a better predictor of discharge disposition than VC or FEV_1 in a population of COPD with very advanced disease, (median VC = 1410 ml, median FEV_1 = 560 l/sec, SA median = 3.2 gm/1000 ml, N = 282) (Fig. 4).[38,84]

The importance of SA, an indicator of nutrition and general health, as a predictor of outcome has been reported by Apelgren et al. in surgical patients[7] and Larca in ventilator patients.[61]

Drugs, Nutrients Interaction and Micronutrients Deficit

The increasingly available wide range of drugs, and multidrug regimens have augmented the possibility of iatrogenic complications. In the treatment of volume overload, fluid and sodium loss should be strictly monitored. Supplementation of vitamins, potassium and magnesium is also usually needed.[93]

Electrolyte disorders can produce impaired respiratory muscle function and several medications have metabolic side effects, or specific pharmacological effects, such as the fatigue enhancing effect of beta blockers or the potential

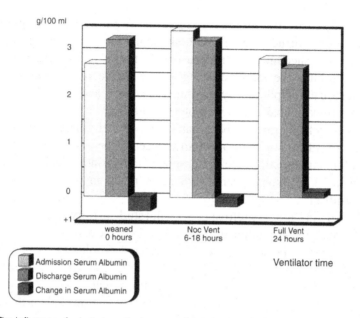

Fig. 2. The influence of admission, discharge and the change of albumin during hospital course on the ventilatory outcome of patients with ventilatory failure.

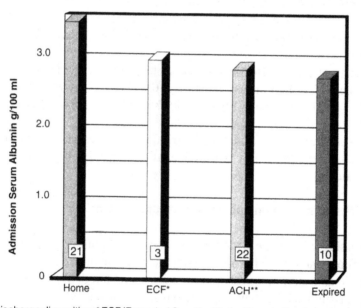

Fig. 3. Discharge disposition: * ECF (Extended Care Facility for Chronic Care); **ACH (Transfer to Acute Hospital because of Complication). Population descriptors: Age = 35 to 85, mean x = 64 years old; length of stay = 1 to 285 days, mean x = 63 days; FEV_1 = 8% to 53%; if = -10 to -58 cm H_2O. Fisher test = Home vs. ACH, p<0.05; Home vs. Expired, p<0.05.

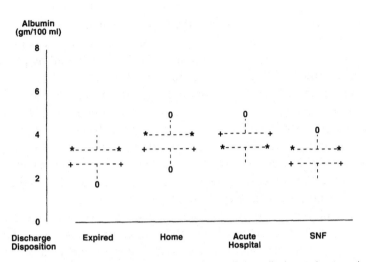

Fig. 4. Differences in admission albumin levels in the four different discharged categories. Acute Hospital = Transfer due to complication: SNF = Skilled Nursing Home for chronic care. (Modified from Roberto M., PHD Dissertation, Yale University, 1989, unpublished)

neuromuscular blockade of calcium channel blockers. These considerations are especially important in patients at risk of ventilator dependency.[29]

Hypophosphatemia - Aubier and associates reported on eight patients with acute respiratory failure and severe hypophosphatemia, which responded to repletion.[14]

Hypocalcemia has also been found to decrease diaphragmatic contractility.[15]

Hypomagnesemia - Malnourished patients and patients with chronic alcoholism are at risk for hypomagnesemia. Magnesium deficiency has been associated with muscle weakness, and potentially with the inability of weaning from the ventilator.[104]

Metabolism and Nutritional Needs in COPD Patients

Patients with increased nutritional needs may be divided into three categories: chronically depleted due to poor intake (starvation), hypermetabolic, hypercatabolic.

Hypermetabolism

The resting energy expenditure (REE) in patients with chronic airflow obstruction is 15% above predicted or 26% above other depleted patients.[48] Up to 71% of COPD patients may lose weight when on a normal or even an above normal diet.[51]

The works of Felig and of Bassill and Dietel have described the difference between starvation in otherwise healthy individuals and the nutritional depletion seen in hypermetabolic-hypercatabolic states like trauma, severe burns, septicemia and severe illness. In starvation, protein catabolism is limited by protein-sparing mechanisms which include the utilization of fat deposits, low levels of insulin, and mobilization of lipolytic enzymes. In hypercatabolic patients, these protein-sparing processes are not operative.[17,18,36,37] Goldstein et al. noted that COPD patients are different from hypermetabolic-hypercatabolic patients, because they can be refed without demonstrating an increased excretion of nitrogen, so while they are hypermetabolic, they are not to be considered hypercatabolic. In fact, emphysema patients can retain 15% on a high-nitrogen and calorie diet similarly to other subjects with no chronic airway obstruction.[47,48]

Wilson et al. found that COPD patients under close supervision, in a metabolic unit, receiving 150 per cent basal metabolic rate calories, using supplementation if needed, can assimilate nutrients and improve respiratory muscle strength.[105] However, refeeding and maintenance of good nutritional status may prove difficult in the advanced COPD with severe malnutrition. At this stage, the motor activity of the ventilatory muscles is greatly stressed, and the mechanical disadvantage of these muscles is augmented by progressive alteration of their resting length and configuration, which adds even more to their work load.

In addition, their chemical environment progressively worsens due to increasing alteration of lung gas exchange. Refeeding, using a high carbohydrate diet, influences ventilatory drive and increases minute ventilation and work of breathing (VE). Increases of the work of breathing are not well tolerated by patients with long term weight loss and end-stage COPD, thus severe nutritional depletion should be prevented in these patients and a low carbohydrate, high-fat diet is recomended to decrease the work of breathing.[6,47,48]

Other factors

Increased ventilatory load in other conditions, such as obesity and pregnancy, does not seem "per se" to cause nutritional depletion. Other factors may play a role in the nutritional depletion of the COPD patients.

Tumor/Necrosis Factor (TNF) has been shown to be a potent inhibitor of lipoprotein lipase and adipogenesis. TNF is a macrophage-derived peptide that has been demonstrated identical to the protein cachectin. Such humoral mechanisms are present in a variety of conditions: sepsis, burns, chronic parasitic infections, shock and heart failure.[21,29,108] They have not been demonstrated yet in COPD.

Recurrent complications, comorbidity. infections, and episodes of cardiorespiratory failure, superimposed on the hypermetabolism of COPD patients, may generate a metabolic bankruptcy difficult to repay even when the episode is resolved.

Decreased blood flow, and any interference with the transport and delivery system of nutrients and oxygen to the ventilatory muscles, especially when they are expected to perform a significantly greater amount of work, will result in impairment of function or injury. Cardiogenic shock, the extreme mechanism of cardiorespiratory perfusion failure, has a very high mortality, and this immediate mortality is markedly and significantly reduced by relieving the work of breathing with assisted mechanical ventilation.[33] Regional variation in blood flow, according to demand, may occur.[81,102]

The biopsy studies of Gertz demonstrated that the reduction in ATP concentration found in the quadricep muscles of COPD patients in respiratory failure, on admission to the Intensive Care, was greater than that found during maximal exertion in healthy subjects, but was compatible with that found in quadricep muscles of patients during cardiogenic shock or severe congestive heart failure or of patients with peripheral occlusive arterial disease.[44]

The swallowing mechanisms in patients with advanced COPD and severe respiratory insufficiency, especially when recovering from respiratory failure, may be impaired, or there may be competition between breathing and swallowing.[38]

Clinical Presentation and Prognosis in COPD and Relationship to Nutritional Status

Weight loss (somatic protein) in COPD patients

Undernutrition in COPD patients is associated with poor prognosis. Mortality is high in underweight COPD patients.[100]

Obesity also contributes to morbidity and mortality, but after episodes of cardiorespiratory failure, patients who were obese and lost excess weight have a better prognosis and longer life expectancy than patients who were underweight.[13] Compared to patients with bronchitis, emphysema patients are more frequently underweight.[73]

Burrows related that in patients with an $FEV_1 > 1.35/l$ the mortality rate over a five year period is not much greater than that of the general population (10-15%). Patients with severe airway obstruction ($FEV_1 < 0.75/l$), poor diffusing capacity (< 50% of predicted) and tachycardia (> 100) showed only a 10% survival after 5 years, but patients with the same FEV_1 who had $CO_2 < 45$ mmHg, better diffusion capacity, and no significant tachycardia had a 40% survival.[27]

Vanderberg reported on a group of COPD patients with hypercapnia ($CO_2 > 45$ mmHg). All patients had a weight loss that exceeded 10%, with an average loss of 20%. In these patients, mortality was significantly higher than in the average population, and cardiopulmonary failure manifested on the average of 21 months after the weight loss was recorded. Importantly, there appeared to be a relationship between dietary intake and the degree of weight loss in these patients.[100]

Nutritional depletion in COPD patients manifests itself first with loss of weight. Weight is not generally a dependable index of malnutrition. Patients can be overweight and malnourished, water retention and lipogenesis may mask nutritional depletion. Children with Kwarshiorkor on a protein poor diet may lose edema, but not show changes in their plasma proteins.[59]

In emphysema patients, however, loss of weight is usually a sign of their hypermetabolism. In these patients monitoring of body weight and early nutritional assessment and intervention are as important as monitoring oxygen saturation and supplementation.

Visceral proteins - In the more advanced stages of COPD, visceral protein depletion becomes more evident. Serum Albumin is a better discriminative indicator of malnutrition, less sensitive to short-term and to contingent dietary and therapeutic interventions than Transferrin or Prealbumin.[8,70,91]

In our hospital, we have found SA to be a good predictor of outcome and discharge disposition in patients with advanced COPD[38,84] (Fig. 4), and in all patients at risk of chronic ventilator dependency (Figs. 2 and 3).

In COPD, Serum Albumin correlates better to hypoxemia and lung diffusing capacity (DLCO), while body weight correlates with VO per cent/kg.[25,91]

Muscle biopsy of COPD patients shows a reduction of Adenosinetriphosphate and Creatine, and other abnormalities regardless of the type and activity levels of skeletal muscle considered and the severity of COPD. Hypoxia and intracellular acidosis were credited with a major role in determining a state of altered cell metabolism.[39]

Gas Exchange, Metabolic and Ventilatory Responses

Hypoxia affects cellular metabolism, structure and function.

Acute hypoxia and hypercapnia increase the chemical drive to ventilation, but may have a negative effect on the ventilatory muscles.[34,56]

Hypoxia induces a three- to sixfold increase in plasma cortisol level due to an increase in the activity of the pituitary gland.[52,74] Glucocorticoids and stress promote preferential muscle wasting and favor visceral glucose and protein production.[42,46]

Hypercapnia augments the noxious effects of hypoxia.[56]

Optimal oxygenation favors anabolism. In underweight patients with emphysema, weight loss often is decreased when they are first placed on oxygen therapy.[78] Quality of life and survival improve in COPD patients on chronic continuous oxygen therapy.[72]

Acute hypercapnia decreases the force-output of the diaphragm for a given level of neural drive both *in vitro* and *in vivo*. This effect is present even with moderate increases in $PaCO_2$ to about 50 mmHg. Hypercapnia decreases diaphragmatic contractility with no change in the diaphragm EMG.[56] Thus, it has been proposed that the effect of hypercapnia is the result of a change in intramuscular pH.

Exercise and nutritional status

Exercise has been found to enhance muscle glycogen synthesis.[22] Due to the increase in the work of breathing in COPD patients one might expect a training effect, but the evidence is that these patients are deconditioned and retraining is beneficial.[55,69,83] Casaburi has proposed anaerobic threshold as a discriminant in training.[28] Specific protocols for inspiratory muscle training have also resulted in improvement of performance.[3,5,20,76,96]

It is known that exercise cannot be abandoned without losing the effects of training. Training should follow established controlled protocols; chronic fatigue, occurring after prolonged periods at submaximal levels, can be associated with minimal injury and inhibit training.[30] Exhaustion is associated with muscle injury.[101] The work of Bellamare and Bigland Ritchie, however, indicates that in humans there is an element of central inhibition which limits the cortical command or the neuromuscular response to it, probably to prevent damage to the diaphragm.[19]

Training of the ventilatory muscles can also benefit neuromuscular conditions, and it has been reported to be beneficial in quadriplegia.[49]

After episodes of acute respiratory failure, the use of appropriate periods of resistive breathing may benefit the patient whose ventilatory muscles have been deconditioned by the use of continuous controlled ventilation and who prove difficult to wean.

Although this can be done even when the patient is not optimally replete,[4] aggressive refeeding should have began and an anabolic state possibly should have been achieved.[59] In order to minimize the need for recurrent ventilator dependency, progression to full weaning may be better done after an optimal possible nutritional status is achieved. Serum albumin is a good prognostic indicator of outcome prognosis [7,38,61,84] (Figs. 2,3,4).

Biopsy studies show that cellular metabolic improvement of respiratory and non-respiratory muscles in these patients is gradual. With refeeding, ventilation, oxygenation, pharmacotherapy and physiotherapy, after one week in the Intensive Care Unit the only improvement noted is in creatine phosphate concentration. With continuing therapy, the ATP concentration returns to values similar to those of control subjects in six to eight weeks. The glycogen values were found not significantly depressed initially and at six to eight weeks were greater than in control subjects.[44]

116

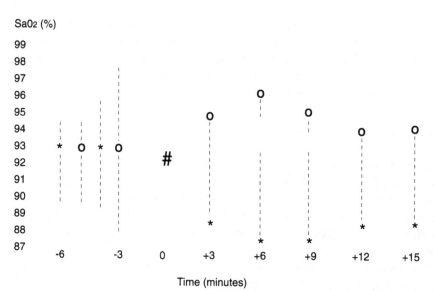

Fig. 5. Prevention of oxygen desaturation by oxymizer during food consumption. ° reservoir cannula; * regular cannula; # onset of food consumption (Brown C., et al., Am. Rev. Respir. Dis., 1988; 137(4) Part 2: 157).

In the rehabilitation regimen of the patient with COPD and respiratory insufficiency, both continuous oxygen and nutritional supplementation are important. Serum albumin has been correlated with exercise performance[92] and oxygen supplementation with increased endurance[103,107] and improved quality of life.

COPD patients who are very breathless to the point of extreme limitation in their activities, when breathing room air, may benefit from oxygen supplement to became independent in the limited activities of daily living.[107]

It is important to protect COPD patients against desaturation not only at rest, but during exertion and sleep and during meals. Demand oxygen delivery systems appear to protect better against desaturation[8,26] and dyspnea,[98,99] and result in improved feeding[38] in COPD patients (Fig. 5). In rehabilitation, the focus often is on optimal transition from the invasive imposed regimen of the acute hospital environment to a simpler one that can be accepted in the longer term.

This often includes not only improvement of function, but when function is definitely lost, then also adjustment to artificial equipment, prescriptions and strategies to allow for function. To gain this acceptance, continuing cooperation between patient, socioeconomic environment and treating team are essential.

There is a need for further assessment and simplifications of dietetic regimens and their interaction with exercise, and ventilation/oxygenation modalities in patients with respiratory insufficiency. Metabolic balance and nutrition, appear no less important than ventilation/oxygenation because these processes are inextricably related.

References

1. Aldrich T.K., Arora N.S., Rochester D.F.: The influence of airway obstruction and respiratory muscle strength on maximal voluntary ventilation in lung disease. Am. Rev. Respir. Dis. 1982; 126: 195-99

2. Aldrich T.K.: The patient at risk of ventilator dependency. Eur. Respir. J. 1989; 7(Supp.): 645

3. Aldrich T.K.: The application of muscle endurance training techniques to the respiratory muscles in COPD. Lung 1985; 163: 15-22

4. Aldrich T.K., Karpel J.P., Ferranti R. et al.: Weaning from mechanical ventilation. Adjunctive use of inspiratory muscle resistive braining. Crit. Care Med. 1989; 17: 2, 143-147

5. Anderson J.B., Dragsted L., Kann T., Johansen S.H. et al.: Resistive breathing training in severe chronic obstructive pulmonary disease. J. Respir. Dis. 1979; 60: 151-156

6. Angelillo V.A., Sukhdarson B., Durfee D., Patterson A.J., O'Donohue W.J.: Effects of low and high carbohydrate feedings in ambulatory patients with chronic obstructive pulmonary disease and chronic hypercapnia. Ann. Intern. Med. 1985; 103 (pt 1): 883-885

7. Apelgen R.N., Rombeau J.T., Twomey P.L., Miller R.A.: Comparison of nutritional indices and outcome in critically ill patients. Crit. Care Med. 1982; 10: 15, 305-307

8. Arlati S., Rolo J., Micaleh E. et al.: A reservoir nasal cannula improves protection given by oxygen during muscular exercise in COPD. Chest 1988; 93: 1165-1169

9. Arora N.S., Rochester D.F.: Respiratory muscle strength and maximal voluntary ventilation in undernourished patients. Am. Rev. Respir. Dis. 1982; 126 (1): 5-8

10. Arora N.S., Rochester D.F.: COPD and human diaphragm muscle dimensions. Chest 1987; 91: 719-724

11. Arora N.S., Rochester D.F.: Effects of general nutritional and muscular status on the human diaphragm. Am. Rev. Respir. Dis. 1977; 115: 84

12. Arora N.S., Rochester D.F.: Effects of body weight and muscularity on human diaphragm muscle mass thickness and area. J. Appl. Physiol. 1982; 52 (1): 64-70

13. Asmundsson T., Kilburn H.: Survival of acute respiratory failure - A study of 239 episodes. Ann. Intern. Med. 1969; 70(3): 471-485

14. Aubier M., Marciano D., Lecocquic Y. et al.: Effect of hypophosphatemia on diaphragm contractility in patients with acute respiratory failure. N. Engl. J. Med. 1985; 313: 420-424

15. Aubier M., Viires N., Piguet J.: Effects of hypocalcemia on diaphragmatic strength generation. J. Appl. Physiol. 1985; 58: 2054-2061

16. Baier H., Samani P.: Ventilatory drive in normal man during semistarvation. Chest 1984; 85(52): 222-225

17. Bassilli H.R., Deitel M.: Effect of nutritional support on weaning patients off mechanical ventilators. J. PEN 1981; 5(2): 161

18. Bassilli H.R., Deitel M.: Nutritional support in long term intensive care with special references to ventilator patients, a review. Can. Anaesth Soc. J. 1981; 28(1): 17

19. Bellamare F., Bigland Ritchie B.: Central components of diaphragmatic fatigue assessed by phrenic nerve stimulation. J. Appl. Phys. 1987; 62: 1307

20. Belman M.J., Mittman C.: Ventilatory muscle training improves exercise capacity in chronic obstructive pulmonary disease patients. Am. Rev. Respir. Dis. 1980; 121: 273-81

21. Beutler B., Cerami A.: Cachectin: more than a tumor necrosis factor. N. Engl. J. Med. 1987; 316: 379

22. Bergstrom J., Hultman F.: Muscle glycogen synthesis after exercise: an enhancing factor localized to the muscle cell in man. Nature 1966; 210: 309-10

23. Bistrian B.R., Blackburn G.L., Scrimshaw N.S., Flatt J.P.: Cellular immunity in semistarved

states in hospitalized adults. Am. J. Clin. Nutr. 1975; 28: 1148-55

24. Braun N.M.T., Rochester D.F.: Muscular weakness and respiratory failure. Am. Rev. Respir. Dis. 1979; 119: 123-125

25. Braun S.R., Keim N.L., Dixon R.M., Clagnaz P., Anderegg A., Shrego E.S.: The prevalence and determinants of nutritional changes in chronic obstructive pulmonary disease. Chest 1984; 86(4): 558-63

26. Brown C. Jr., Ferranti R.D., Sparapani M.: Reservoir nasal cannula prevents desaturation in COPD patients during eating. Am. Rev. Respir. Dis. 1988; 137(4) Part 2: 157

27. Burrows B., Earle R.H.: Care and properties of chronic obstructive lung disease. N. Engl. J. Med. 1969; 280: 397

28. Casaburi R., Wasserman K., Potessio A. et al.: A new perspective in pulmonary rehabilitation: anaerobic threshold as a discriminant in training. Eur. Respir. J. 1989; 7 (suppl): 618S-623S

29. Clowes GHA J., George B.C., Villee C.A. Jr., et al.: Muscle proteolysis induced by a circulating peptide in patients with sepsis or trauma. N. Engl. J. Med. 1983; 308: 545-552

30. Davis K.J.A., Packer L., Brooks G.A.: Biochemical adaptation of mitochondria, muscle, and whole animal respiration to endurance training. Arch. Biochem. Biophys. 1981; 209: 539-554

31. Demey H.E., Van Merbeck J.P., Vanderwonde F.F.T., Prove A.M., Martin J.J., Bossaert L.L.: Respiratory insufficiency in acid maltase deficiency. The effect of high protein diet. J. Parenter. Enteral Nutr. 1989; 13: 3, 321-323

32. Doekel R.C., Zwillic C.W., Scoggings C.H., Kryger M., Weil J.V.: Clinical semi-starvation: depression of hypoxic ventilatory response. N. Engl. J. Med. 1976; 295: 358-61

33. Dubier M., Trippenbach T., Roussos C.: Respiratory muscle fatigue during cardiogenic shock. J. Appl. Physiol. 1981; 51: 499

34. Farkas G., Prefant C. et al.: The failing inspiratory muscles under normoxic and hypoxic conditions. Am. Rev. Respir. Dis. 1981; 124: 274-9

35. Farkas G.A., Roussos C.: Adaptability of the hamster diaphragm to exercise and or emphysema. J. Appl. Physiol. 1982; 53(5): 1263-72

36. Felig P.: Starvation. In: DeGrott L.J. (Ed.) Endocrinology. New York, Grune & Stratton, 1979; 3: 1927

37. Felig P., Havel R.J., Smith L.H. Jr.: Metabolism and Nutrition. New York, McGraw-Hill, 1981; 548-582

38. Ferranti R.D., Roberto M., Brown C. Jr., Coehlo C.: Oral intake, O_2, dyspnea, dysphagia and other considerations in COPD patients. In: Ferranti R.D. (Ed.) Nutrition and Ventilatory Function - Current Topics in Rehabilition. Verona, Bi & Gi Publishers, London, Springer Verlag, 1992; 181-189

39. Fiaccadori E., Del Canale S., Guariglia A.: Nutritional and metabolic aspects of COPD in rehabilitation muscles. In: A. Grassino (Ed.) Respiratory Muscles in Chronic Obstructive Pulmonary Disease - Current Topics in Rehabilitation. Verona, Bi & Gi Publishers, London, Springer-Verlag; 1988, 111-123

40. Gail D.B., Massaro G.D., Massaro D.: Influence of fasting on the lung. J. Appl. Physiol. 1977; 42(1): 88-92

41. Garbagni R., Coppo F., Grassini G., Cardillino G.: Effects of lipid loading and fasting on pulmonary function in respiration. 1968; 25: 458-64

42. Gardiner P.F., Montano G., Simpson D.R. et al.: Effects of glucocorticoids treatment and food restriction on rat limb muscles. Am. J. Physiol. 1980; 238 (Endocrin. Metab. 1): E124-E130

43. Gardiner P.F., Hill B., Simpson D.R. et al.: Effect of mild weight-lifting program on the prognosis of glucocorticoid induced atrophy. Pflugers Arch. 1980; 385: 147-153

44. Gertz I., Hendstierna G., Hellers G., Wahren J.: Muscle metabolism in patients with chronic

obstructive lung disease and acute respiratory failure. Clin. Sci. Mol. Med. 1977; 52: 395-403

45. Gibson G.I., Pride N.B., Davis J.N., Loh L.C.: Pulmonary mechanics in patients with respiratory muscle weakness. Am. Rev. Respir. Dis. 1977; 115(3): 389-95

46. Goldberg A.L.: Influence of insulin and contractile activity on muscle and protein balance. Diabetes 1979; 28 (suppl): 18-29

47. Goldstein S.A., Thomashow B.M., Kretan V., Askanazi J., Kinney J.M., Elwin D.H.: Nitrogen and energy relationships in malnourished patients with emphysema. Am. Rev. Respir. Dis. 1989; 138(3): 636-44

48. Goldstein S.A., Askanazi J.: Macronutrients effect on metabolism and ventilation in patients with chronic lung disease. In: Ferranti R.D. (Ed.) *Nutrition and Ventilatory Function* - Current Topics in Rehabilitation. Verona, Bi & Gi Publishers, London, Springer -Verlag, 1992; 167-173

49. Gross D., Ladd H.W., Riley E.J., MacKlem P.T., Grassino A.: The effect of training on strength and endurance of the diaphragm in quadriplegia. Am. J. Med. 1980; 68: 27-35

50. Gross I., Rooney S.A., Warshaw J.P.: The inhibition of enzymes related to pulmonary fatty acid and phospholipid synthesis by dietary deprivation in the rat. Biochem. Biophys. Res. Commun. 1975; 64: 69

51. Hunter A.M.B., Casey M.A., Larsh H.W.: The nutritional status of patients with chronic obstructive pulmonary disease. Am. Rev. Respir. Dis. 1967; 95: 556-566

52. Hyes M.P., Farber M.O., Manfredi F.: Acute effects of hypoxia on renal and endocrine function in normal humans. Am. J. Physiol. 1982; 243(3): R 265-270

53. Iannuzzo C.D., Noble E.G., Hamilton N., Dabroki B.: Effects of streptozotocin diabetes, insulin treatment, and training on the diaphragm. J. Appl. Physiol. 1982; 52(6): 1471-1475

54. Ivy J.L., Costill D.L., Maxwell B.D.: Skeletal muscle determinants of maximum aerobic power in man. Eur. J. Appl. Physiol. 1971; 315-25

55. Jones N.L., Berman L.E., Barkiewicz P.D. et al.: Chronic obstructive respiratory disorders. In: Skinner J. (Ed.) *Exercise Testing and Prescription for Special Cases*. Philadelphia, Lea & Febiger, 1977; 175-188

56. Juan G., Calverley P., Talamo C.: Effect of carbon dioxide on diaphragmatic function in human beings. N. Engl. J. Med. 1984; 310: 874-9

57. Kelsen S.G., Ference M., Kapoor S.: Effects of prolonged undernutrition on structure and function of the diaphragm. J. Appl. Physiol. 1985; 58: 1354-9

58. Kelsen S.: The effects of undernutrition on the respiratory muscles. Clin. Chest Med. 1986; 7(4): 100-101

59. Kinney J.M., Weissman C.: Forms of malnutrition in stressed and unstressed patients. Clin. Chest Med. 1986; 7: 101-110

60. Kubista V., Kiston J., Pette D.: Thyroid hormone induced changes in the enzyme activity pattern of energy supplying metabolism of fast (white), slow (red) and heart muscle. Eur. J. Biomed. 1971; 18: 553-560

61. Larca L., Greenbaum D.M.: Effectiveness of intensive nutritional regimens in patients who fail to wean from mechanical ventilation. 1982; 10: 297-300

62. Lange P., Groth S., Mortensen J. et al.: Diabetes mellitus, plasma glucose and lung function in a cross sectional population study. Eur. Respir. J. 1989; 2: 14

63. Law D.K., Dudrick S.J., Abdou N.I.: Immunocompetence of patients with protein-caloric malnutrition. Ann Intern. Med. 1973; 79: 545-550

64. Layzer R.B., Havel R.J., McElroy M.B.: Partial deficiency of carnitine palmityl transferase: physiologic and biochemical consequences. Neurology 1980; 30: 627-33

65. Lewis M.I., Sieck G.C., Fournier M., Belman M.J.: Effect of nutritional deprivation on diaphragm contractility and muscle fiber size. J. Appl. Physiol. 1988; 60: 596-603

66. Lewis M.I., Belman M.J.: Nutrition and the respiratory muscles. Clin. Chest Med. 1988; 9(2): 337-48

67. Malloy D.W., Dhingra G., Solven F.S.: Hypomagnesemia and respiratory muscle power. Am. Rev. Respir. Dis. 1984; 129: 497-498

68. Mayer M., Rosen F.: Interaction of glucocorticoids and androgens with skeletal muscle. Metabolism 1977; 26: 937-962

69. McGavin C.R., Gupta S.P., Lloyd E.L. et al.: Physical rehabilitation for the chronic bronchitic. Results of a controlled trial of exercise in the home. Thorax 1977; 32: 307-311

70. Mobarhan S.: The role of albumin in nutritional support. J. Am. Coll. Nutr. 1988; 7: 445-52

71. Niederman M.S., Merrill W.W., Ferranti R.D., Pagano K.M., Palmer L.B., Reynolds H.Y.: Nutritional status and bacterial binding in the lower respiration tract in patients with chronic tracheostomy. Ann. Intern. Med. 1984; 100: 795-800

72. Nocturnal oxygen therapy trial group. Continuous or nocturnal oxygen therapy in hypoxemic chronic obstructive pulmonary disease. Ann. Intern. Med. 1980; 93: 391-398

73. Openbier D.R.: Nutritional status and lung function in patients with chronic obstructive lung disease. Am. Rev. Respir. Dis. 1981; 124: 376

74. Ou L.C., Tenney S.M.: Adrenocortical function in rats chronically exposed to high altitude. J. Appl. Physiol. 1979; 47: 1185-1187

75. Pain V.M., Albertse E.C., Garlick P.J.: Protein metabolism in skeletal muscle diaphragm and heart of diabetic rats. Am. J. Physiol. 1983; 245: E604-E610

76. Pardy R.L., Rivington R.N., Despas P.J., Macklem P.T.: The effect of inspiratory muscle training in exercise performance in chronic airflow limitation. Am. Rev. Respir. Dis. 1981; 123: 426-33

77. Pernow B.B., Havel R.J., Jennings D.B.: The second wind phenomena in McArdle syndrome. Acta Med. Scand. Suppl. 1967; 472: 294-307

78. Petty T., Finigan M.: Clinical evaluation of prolonged oxygen therapy in chronic airway obstruction. A.M.T. 1968; 45: 242-252

79. Primlack R.A., Whincup G., Tsanakas J.N., Milner R.D.: Reduced vital capacity in insulin-dependent diabetes. Diabetes 1987; 36: 32-45

80. Raff H.: Vasopressin, ACTH and corticosteroids during hypercapnia and graded hypoxia in dogs. Am. J. Physiol. 1983; 244: E 453-E458

81. Reid M.B., Johnson R.L. Jr.: Efficiency, maximal blood flow, and aerobic work capacity of canine diaphragm. J. Appl. Physiol. 1983; 54: 763-72

82. Renzetti A.D., McClement J.H.: The Veterans Administration cooperative study of pulmonary function: morbidity in relation to respiratory function in chronic pulmonary disease. Am. J. Med. 1966; 41: 115-129

83. Ries A.L., Archibald C.J.: Endurance and exercise training at maximal targets in patients with COPD. J. Cardiopulmonary Rehab. 1987; 7: 594-601

84. Roberto M.: *Predictors of Outcome in COPD.* Yale University, 1989, unpublished

85. Rochester D.F., Braun N.M.T., Arora N.S.: Respiratory muscle strength in chronic obstructive lung disease. Am. Rev. Respir. Dis. 1979; 119: 151-154

86. Rochester D.F., Braun N.M.T.: Determinants of maximal inspiratory pressure in chronic obstructive pulmonary disease. Am. Rev. Respir. Dis. 1985; 132: 42-47

87. Rosenbaum S.H., Askanazi A.L.: Respiratory patterns in profound nutritional depletion (abstract). Anesthesiology 1979; 51: 5366

88. Roza A.M., Twitt D., Shizgal H.M.: Transferrin, a poor measure of nutritional status. J. Penn. 1984; 8: 523-28

89. Sahebjami H., Vassallo C.L., Wirman J.A.: Lung mechanics and ultrastructure in prolonged starvation. Am. Rev. Respir. Dis. 1978; 177: 77-83

90. Sahebjami H., Wirman J.A.: Emphysema-like changes in the lungs of straved rats. Am. Rev. Respir. Dis. 1981; 124 (5): 619-24

91. Schols A., Mostert R., Soeters P., Greve L.H., Wouters E.F.: Inventory of nutritional status in patients with COPD. Chest 1989; 96: 247-9

92. Schols A., Mostert R., Soeters P.: Nutritional status and exercise performance in patients with chronic obstructive lung disease. Thorax 1989; 44: 937-941

93. Scifferdecker C., Driscoll D.F., Bistrian R.B.: Management guidelines when drugs and nutrients interact. J. Crit. Illness 1990; 5(1): 34-41

94. Sheldon G.F., Petersen S.R.: Malnutrition and cardiopulmonary function. J. Parent. Enteral Nutr. 1980; 4: 376-383

95. Sirizisma S., Suskind R., Edelman R., Asvapaka C., Olson R.E.: Secretory and serum IgA in children with protein calorie malnutrition. Pediatrics 1975; 55: 166

96. Sonne L.J., Davis A.J.: Increased exercise performance in patients with severe COPD following inspiratory training. Chest 1982; 81: 436-439

97. Suspinki G.S., Lelren S.G.: Effect of elastic-induced emphysema on the force generating ability of the diaphragm. J. Clin. Invest. 1982; 70: 978-988

98. Tiep B.L., Christofer K.L., Spofford B.T. et al.: Pulsed conserving devices. Respir. Care 1985; 30: 833

99. Tiep B.L., Christofer K.L., Spofford B.T. et al.: Pulsed normal and transtracheal oxygen delivery. Chest 1990; 97: 2

100. Vanderberg F., Van de Woestine K.P., Gyselen A.: Weight changes in the terminal stages of chronic obstructive lung disease. Am. Rev. Respir. Dis. 1967; 95: 556-66

101. Vihko V., Salminen A. et al.: Exhaustive exercise, endurance training, and acid hydrolase activity in skeletal muscle. J. Appl. Physiol. 1979; 47: 43-50

102. Viires N., Sillye G., Gaddes G., Aubier M., Rassidakis A., Roussos C.: Regional blood flow distribution in dog during induced hypotension and low cardiac output. J. Clin. Invest. 1983; 72(3): 935-67

103. Vjas M.N., Banister J.W., Morton S. et al.: Response to exercise in patients with chronic airway destruction: effects of breathing 40% oxygen. Am. Rev. Respir. Dis. 1972; 103: 401-412

104. Whang R., Rydeck P.: Frequency of hypomagnesemia and hypermagnesemia. JAMA 1990; 263(22): 3063

105. Wilson D.O., Rogers R.M., Sanders M.H. et al.: Nutritional intervention in undernourished patients with emphysema. Am. Rev. Respir. Dis. 1986; 134: 672-677

106. Winick M.: *Hunger Disease: Studies by the Jewish Physicians in the Warsaw Ghetto.* New York, Wiley and Sons, 1979

107. Woodcock A.A., Gross E.R., Geddes D.M.: Oxygen relieves breathlessness in "Pink Puffers". Lancet 1981; 907

108. Fong F., Lowry F.S., Cerami A.: Cachetin/TNF: a macrophage protein that induces cachexia and shock. JPEN 12: 46, Suppl. 72s-75s

12. The Right Heart in Precapillary Pulmonary Hypertension: Pathophysiological and Therapeutic Aspects

M. MORPURGO

Department of Cardiology, San Carlo Borromeo Hospital, Milan, Italy

Pulmonary heart disease begins with pulmonary hypertension (PH) and ends in right ventricular (RV) failure - although, as we shall see later in detail, PH is by no means the only factor involved. In this presentation we shall discuss only the two intermediate stages of pulmonary heart disease, namely RV enlargement and RV dysfunction (Fig. 1).

We shall take as our starting point the critical review "Evaluation of Right Ventricular Function: Controversies and Methods of Investigation", presented by Dr Jezek and myself at the International Symposium "Pulmonary Circulation V" (Prague 1989).[30] In that paper we listed several circumstances that made the assessment of RV function a tough proposition, as follows:

1. the right heart is a structure subject to continuous change in terms of pressure, flow rates and shape;
2. the RV pumps blood into a vascular bed likewise subject to changes in size and geometry;
3. the RV and pulmonary vasculature influence each other in a ceaseless interplay (ventricular-arterial coupling, or matching);
4. the RV is continuously assisted by the left ventricle.

Today we will try to update our 1989 critical review by discussing some recent contributions to the assessment of RV function with special attention to diastolic function, and adding a short section on therapeutics, as suggested by this workshop's organizers. Methods for assessing RV systolic function in terms of regional RV contraction abnormalities have been developed.[12] According to Ratner et al.[24]

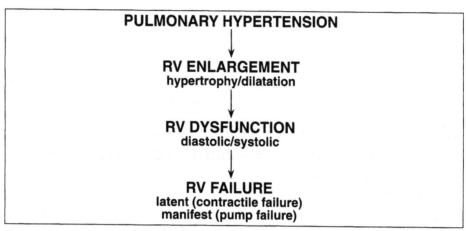

PULMONARY HYPERTENSION

↓

RV ENLARGEMENT
hypertrophy/dilatation

↓

RV DYSFUNCTION
diastolic/systolic

↓

RV FAILURE
latent (contractile failure)
manifest (pump failure)

Fig. 1

the frequent detection of RV wall motion abnormalities in patients with normal RV volume and total ejection fraction suggests that subclinical dysfunction of this chamber could be assessed quite easily by a radionuclide angiography method utilizing five RV chords to explore regional wall motion. Abbott and his associates[1] determine RV systolic performance by a combination of rest and peak exercise cine-computed tomograms (CT) and Doppler echocardiography, the two methods seemingly affording finer analysis of RV function. In Abbott's experience the so-called RV "contractility index" (being the ratio of end-systolic pressure to volume) was significantly higher in lung disease with PH than in normal subjects, despite a reduced RV ejection fraction.

This finding is in strikingly good agreement both with ancient clinical observations[5] and with the results published in recent papers.[4,17] Burghuber and Bergmann noted that even in the presence of a decreased RV ejection fraction, overall RV function (expressed in terms of stroke volume index and cardiac index) as well as RV "contractility" (expressed as P/V ratio) were well preserved in chronic obstructive pulmonary disease (COPD) with PH.

Still, recent literature[13,25] makes us aware of certain limitations in the measurement of the P/V relationship - as we ourselves mentioned in our critical review (Tab. I).

And furthermore, from a conceptual point of view, we must make a distinction between what the heart muscle is capable of doing and what it actually does in a given situation, such as a state of pressure overload.[19] Capability, or the potential for contraction that the muscle commands by virtue of local physicochemical conditions, has come to be called "contractility"; actual performance, however, also reflects the limitations imposed by external mechanical circumstances on the heart muscle's ability to respond. So far, no satisfactory operational definition of myocardial contractility has been forthcoming - the only certain thing is that such

Table I. Limits of P/V relation measurements.

- Not always linear	(M.I.M. Noble, 1988)
- Not independent of loading conditions	(Redington et al., 1990)*
- Not independent of host size	(Maugham and Oikawa, 1989)
- Sensitive to changes in ventricular compliance	(W.W. Parmley, 1985)
- RV end-ejection and end-systole do not coincide	(Sagawa et al., 1985)
- Difficulty of accurate measurements of RV volumes	(Sagawa et al., 1985)
- Need of two or more P/V loops	(R.K. Albert, 1988)

a parameter cannot be expressed by a single numerical value or simple ratio. As Blinks and Jewell pointed out in 1972, "if the index is really simple, its informational content is unlikely to be adequate". The central point is that cardiac work inevitably depends both on myocardial contractility and on ventricular load, and the effects of these two factors are hard to identify separately.[19]

Coming now to RV diastolic function we may start by recalling that the diastolic period consists of various phases, namely protodiastole, isovolumic relaxation, rapid filling, passive filling, and atrial contraction. When doctors speak of diastolic dysfunction it is not always clear which component of diastole they refer to.[23]

In fact, ventricular diastolic function is a complex process, and the phrase "diastolic dysfunction" has come to include changes in everything, from fundamental myocardial properties to alterations in loading conditions.[11,27]

Ventricular diastole is affected by a number of interacting and often confusing variables such as age, the heart rate, preload conditions, and the asynchronous wall motion during relaxation seen in hypertrophic ventricles.[11] Pressure overload hypertrophy is associated with beneficial as well as detrimental features (Tab. II).[16]

Table II. Pressure overload hypertrophy.

Beneficial aspects:
- increases ventricular work
- normalizes wall stress
- normalizes systolic shortening

Detrimental aspects:
- decreases diastolic distensibility
- impairs ventricular relaxation
- impairs coronary vasodilator reserve

B.H. Lorell, W. Grossman[16]

The progressive loss of ventricular distensibility during diastole is revealed by a substantial increase of ventricular filling pressure relative to diastolic volume. In the case of the RV, filling characteristics are reflected by the flow velocity curve through the tricuspid valve - unfortunately, diastolic flow velocities at that level are technically more difficult to measure than those of the mitral valve.[19]

Ideally, a complete analysis of diastolic function should include an estimate of chamber stiffness (being the ratio of diastolic ventricular pressure to ventricular volume), myocardial stiffness (diastolic stress/strain relationship), end-diastolic volume, and myocardial muscle mass.[27]

Currently, overall diastolic function is assessed chiefly by combined measurements of deceleration time and of the isovolumic relaxation period.[20]

Patients with RV hypertrophy due to chronic pressure overload and reduced RV compliance may show a prolongation of deceleration time (time from peak filling to baseline extrapolation of velocity decline); a decrease of E/A ratio (early-to-late diastolic filling); and abnormal venous inflow velocities.[20] It should be borne in mind, at any rate, that nonuniformity of ventricular relaxation affects the measurements of diastolic function quite dramatically.

The most common pathology that underlies impaired ventricular distensibility is interstitial fibrosis of the heart muscle.[14]

In that respect, several lines of evidence suggest the possibility of modifying the matrix of interstitial proteins with suitable drugs, thereby materially influencing the passive properties of the myocardium. In cardiac pressure overload hypertrophy the collagen quota of the myocardium relative to muscle is increased, and this is associated with changes in collagen structures. Although collagen content persists after the normalization of PAP in chronically hypoxic rats,[21] appropriate drug treatment might alter the nature or extent of changes in extracellular proteins and modify the passive pressure/volume relationship of the hypertrophic myocardium.[11]

From a practical point of view certain calcium entry blockers (verapamil) or beta adrenergic blockers, all being drugs with negative inotropic properties, may worsen the condition of patients with systolic ventricular failure while improving that of patients with diastolic dysfunction.

Drugs that increase cyclic AMP, like milrinone (a phosphodiesterase inhibitor) and forskolin (a direct activator of adenylate cyclase), may improve diastolic function.[14] According to Packer[22] there is no excluding that part of the improvement seen with vasodilatator and inotropic drug treatment in heart failure reflects the effects of such drugs on diastolic performance. Certainly the beneficial partial-agonist effect of xamoterol on diastolic function, along with the alleviation of tachycardia during maximum exercise, allows better RV filling.[18]

Digitalis does not improve diastolic function, in fact it may theoretically make it worse by increasing the consumption of energy associated with augmented inotropy, at the same time depleting energy stores needed for diastolic relaxation.[27]

And in patients with PH secondary to COPD, digitalis is probably of no use since RV systolic performance is not impaired.[2] As mentioned at the start, when we consider the possible cause of right heart dysfunction in patients with chronic lung disease and PH we must not assume that the elevated pulmonary artery pressure is the only factor at play.[6]

What other factors can increase RV afterload? To answer that question we must recall that RV afterload is expressed more accurately by pulmonary input impedance (PII) than by pulmonary vascular resistance (PVR) as usually calculated. Whereas the traditional concept of PVR makes no allowance for the pulsatile character of pulmonary blood flow, PII does just that, since it represents the ratio of oscillatory flow to oscillatory pressure.

The relationship between pressure and flow is a complex affair, not only on account of the intermittent pattern of ventricular ejection but also in view of the elastic properties of the proximal pulmonary arteries. Actually, changes in the mechanical properties of the pulmonary Windkessel have profound repercussions both on the phase and on the amplitude of the pressure/flow ratio, and also on overall RV performance, in the setting of what has been called "ventricular-arterial coupling"[19] or "ventricular-arterial matching".[12] Arterial stiffness and the loss of compliance associated with PH reduce the cushion-like mode of pulsing ventricular ejection and so lead to hydraulic ventricular wall load stress with adverse effects on myocardial oxygen consumption. Furthermore, these changes contribute to the maintenance of high levels of PAP, signally of systolic PAP.

For this situation Robin[26] cogently remarked that "Pulmonary hypertension begets additional pulmonary hypertension". In patients with PH, on the other hand, oxygen breathing may reduce the stiffness of main pulmonary arteries.[15]

Back to our search for possible factors that may increase RV afterload in addition to PH itself, we may wonder if a difference between the "true" pulsatile PII and cardiac load as calculated conventionally from PAP and cardiac output measurements is enough to account for the presence of RV dysfunction even at the low pressure usually found in COPD patients. The question was brought up by J. Butler,[6] who also suggested as a further possibility that external impedance to RV function might be present in the "cardiac fossa";[6] in that respect, distended lower lobes with tense pleural surfaces might be partly to blame.

Another factor to be considered in COPD patients is coughing. As stated by Uhlenbruck many years ago,[28] "Coughing and the associated sudden increase in intrathoracic pressure in the long run impose an important strain on the right heart. Coughing hinders diastolic filling".

As said before, RV systolic function is apparently normal in most patients with PH secondary to chronic lung disease; and some drugs, like xamoterol, may at least theoretically alleviate diastolic dysfunction if such be present. Following are some tentative therapeutic suggestions, offered with an eye on the known interactions between the heart and the pulmonary vasculature. For oxygen therapy you may want to see a number of recent critical reviews on the subject, only bear in mind that, aside from its complex action on pulmonary vessels, oxygen therapy may have some important effects on myocardial metabolism.

In cardiac failure, functional impairment depends not only on anatomical and biochemical changes in the heart but also on the extent of compensatory adjustments for cardiac dysfunction: exercise tolerance is as dependent on peripheral circulation as it is on cardiac reserve.[29]

Could this concept, generally applied to the peripheral circulation, be valid for the pulmonary circulation as well? We know, for instance, that the vasodilation reserve of peripheral vessels during exercise is curtailed in heart failure patients, and we may want to argue that the reduced distensibility of the pulmonary vasculature might have similar effect in patients with PH of long standing.

Further: the increase of exercise capacity obtained with diuretics despite a reduced cardiac output has been attributed to an improvement of vascular reactivity due to reduction of the sodium content of vascular walls.[10]

Could the same hypothesis be extended to pulmonary vessels, particularly in hypoxic PH? Working with rats and isolated small pulmonary arteries, some authors[31] found that with developing chronic pulmonary hypoxia the vascular smooth musculature shows gradual hyperpolarization associated with increased activity of the electrogenic Na^+, K^+ pump.

Indapamide is known to reduce intracellular calcium and phosphate ion levels that may be involved in arterial rigidity.

We may figure that the combination of binding to elastin and a reduced calcium and phosphate uptake into smooth muscle might reduce the arterial rigidity seen in hypertensive patients.[8] And since indapamide also stimulates the production of vasodilatator and inhibits the synthesis of vasoconstrictor prostanoids, don't you think that this drug should be tested in patients with pulmonary hypertension?

Note that we have deliberately ignored the β_2-agonists salbutamol, pirbuterol and terbutaline. The fact is that these drugs did increase RVEF, RV stroke work index and cardiac output and reduce PVR in acute trials on patients with COPD and PH; but the experience accruing from trials of other putative pulmonary vasodilators discourages the hope of achieving long-lasting benefits with β_2-agonists.

For instance, a recent study by Biernacki et al.[3] shows that the beneficial effects of oral pirbuterol on cardiac output, PVR and RVEF are no longer detectable after 6 months of continuing treatment. To conclude: our Prague report contained a few recommendations such as:

a. Avoid the term "contractility" when you are actually assessing pump performance.
b. Bear in mind that ventricular pump function may appear normal if loading conditions are favorable.

c. Do not apply measurements or indices to the RV simply because they were good for the left heart.

d. Consider RV function as a whole rather than in terms of separate measurements.

In the matter of treating RV dysfunction in patients with pulmonary hypertension, we are inclined to swing from the traditional approach targeted on the remote and terminal consequences of right heart failure to a more modern, as yet speculative, and possibly premature attitude that takes into account all the mechanical, humoral and biochemical factors conducive to RV dysfunction in PH patients.

References

1. Abbott J.A., Himelman R.B., Elan D., Scheinman B.A., Wan T.: Right ventricular performance in lung disease. JACC 1990; 15: 161(abstr.)
2. Berglund E.: Hemodynamics of the right ventricle in chronic lung disease Bull. Physiopathol. Respir. 1972; 8: 1417-1422
3. Biernacki W., Prince K., Whyte K., MacNee W., Flenley D.C.: The effects of six months of daily treatment with β-2 agonist oral pirbuterol on pulmonary hemodynamics in patients with chronic hypoxic cor pulmonale receiving longterm oxygen therapy. Am. Rev. Respir. Dis. 1989; 139: 492-497
4. Burghuber O.C., Bergmann H.: Right ventricular contractility in chronic obstructive pulmonary disease. A combined radionuclide and hemodynamic study. Respiration 1988; 53: 1-12
5. Burns A.: Osservazioni sopra alcune piu frequenti ed importanti malattie del cuore, sull'aneurisma dell'arco dell'aorta e sulla non naturale pulsazione nella regione epigastrica. Milano Bucher, 1816
6. Butler J.: Cor pulmonale. In: J.F.Murray, J.A. Nadel (Eds.) Textbook of Respiratory Medicine. Philadelphia, Saunders, 1988; 1410
7. Butler J.: The heart is not always in good hands. Chest 1990; 97: 453-460
8. Campbell D.B., Brackman F.: Cardiovascular protective properties of indapamide. Am. J. Cardiol. 1990; 65: 11H-27H
9. Chakko S., de Marchena E., Kessler KM., Masterson B.J., Myerburg R.J.: Right ventricular diastolic function in systemic hypertension. Am. J. Cardiol. 1990; 65: 1117-1120
10. Cohen-Solal A.: Improving exercise tolerance in patients with heart failure: should we treat the heart or the periphery? Eur. Heart. J. 1989; 10: 866-871
11. Covell J.W.: Factor influencing diastolic function. Possible role of the extracellular matrix, Circulation 1990; 81 (suppl III): 155-158
12. Elzinga G., Toorp G.P., Gross D.R., Westerhof N.: Geometry and pump function in cardiac ventricular hypertrophy. Am. J. Cardiol. 1990; 65: 23G-29G
12. Ferlinz J.: Right ventricular performance assays: slowly coming of age. JACC 1989; 13: 360-362
13. Foult J.M., Loiseau A., Nitenberg A.: Size dependence of the end-systolic stress/volume ratio in humans: implications for the evaluation of myocardial contractile performance in pressure and volume overload. JACC 1990; 16: 124-129
14. Grossman W. Diastolic dysfunction and congestive heart failure. Circulation 1990; 81 (suppl III) 1-7
15. Haneda T., Nakajima T., Shirato K., Onodera S., Takishima T.: Effects of oxygen breathing on pulmonary vascular input impedance in patients with pulmonary hypertension. Chest 1983; 83: 520-527

16. Lorell B.H., Grossman W.: Cardiac hypertrophy:the consequences for diastole. JACC 1987; 9: 1189-1193

17. MacNee W., Wathen C.G., Flenley D.C., Muir A.D.: The effects of control led oxygen therapy on ventricular function in patients with stable and decompensated cor pulmonale. Am. Rev. Respir. Dis. 1988; 137: 1289-1295

18. Marlow H.F.: Review of clinical experience with xamoterol. Circulation 1990; 81 (suppl III): 93-98

19. Milnor W.R.: *Hemodynamics*, 2 ed., Baltimore, Williams and Wilkins, 1989; 267

20. Nishimura R.A., Abel M.D., Hatle L.K., Taik A.J.: Assessment of diastolic function of the heart: background and current applications of Doppler echocardiography. Part II. Clinical studies. Mayo Clin. Proc. 1989; 64: 181-204

21. Ostadal B., Pelouch V., Kolar F., Prochazka I., Cihak R., Widimski I.: Experimental right ventricular hypertrophy, Intern. Symp Pulmonary Circulation V, Prague 1989; 108 (abstr.)

22. Packer M.: Diastolic function as a target of therapeutic interventions in chronic heart failure. Eur. Heart J. 1990; 11 (suppl C): 35-40

23. Poole-Wilson P.A.: Introduction to the Satellite Symposium to the XIth Congress of the European Society of Cardiology "Heart failure and diastolic dysfunction - new insights" Eur. J. Cardiol. 1990; 11(suppl C): 1

24. Ratner S.C., Por J. Huang, Friedman M.I., Pierson R.N.: Assessment of right ventricular anatomy and function by quantitative radionuclide ventriculography. JACC 1989; 13: 354-359

25. Redington A.N., Rigby M.L., Shinebourne E.A., Oldershaw P.J.: Changes in the pressure/volume relation of the right ventricle when its loading conditions are modified. Br. Heart J. 1990; 63: 45-49

26. Robin E.D.: Some basic and clinical challenges in the pulmonary circulation. Chest 1982; 81: 357-362

27. Shub C.: Heart failure and abnormal ventricular function. Pathophysiology and clinical correlation (part 2). Chest 1989; 96: 906-914

28. Uhlenbruck P.: *Die Herzkrankheiten*. Leipzig, J.A. Barth Verlag, 1949; 240

29. Wasserman K. Measures of functional capacity in patients with heart failure. Circulation 1990; 81 (suppl II): 1-4

30. Jezeck V., Morpurgo M.: Right heart failure in chroniclung disease. Where are we now? In: Jezeck V., Morpurgo M., Tramarin R. (Eds.): *Right Ventricular Hypertrophy and Function in Chronic Lung Disease*. Verona, Bi & Gi Publishers, London Springer Verlag, 1992, 1-9

31. Altura J.: Pharmacology of the pulmonary circulation: an overview. In: J.A. Will et al. (Eds.) *The Pulmonary Circulation in Health and Disease*. Orlando, Academic Press, 1987; 85

13. Dismission Criteria from Intensive Care Unit

J.F. MUIR

Service de Pneumologie, Hôpital de Bois-Guillaume, CHU Rouen, France

The decision to discharge a patient out of the intensive care unit is different to take with chronic respiratory insufficiency (CRI) versus other types of acute disorders. Frequently, the CRI patient is authorized to leave the intensive care unit when his dependency to the respirator has not disappeared, and it will be necessary to wait during a new period devoted to a weaning procedure before getting home. Thus, in CRI patients, the decision is governed by the possibilities for the patient to return to home as soon as possible,[1] which will be possible if the extrarespiratory status appears stable, and if the weaning procedure has been either completed or stopped to a reasonable level considering the availability of home ventilation.

Whatever the etiology of the CRI, the first step is to obtain a control of the precipitating factors of the acute respiratory failure (ARF) episode (infection), and a stabilization of the general extrarespiratory conditions (hemodynamic status) which are often impaired before, during and after the ARF episode.[2]

These actions are involved in the preweaning period, weaning itself being impossible if the general status of the patient has not been previously improved.

Three conditions may be seen during and after the weaning trials.

1. The patient appears impossible to wean, at least during a short period of time:

If the extrarespiratory status is controlled, and if the patient feels well under the continuous ventilatory support, it is possible to discharge him from the ICU to a "chronic ventilatory care unit",[3] where he will be educated as well as his family to his future life-long home stay under continuous mechanical ventilation with tracheostomy. That case is commonly managed in post-neurosurgical patients with head and neck injury, but also in patients with neuromuscular disease. We must remember also that home mechanical ventilation (HMV) was born with CRI secondary to poliomyelitis.

2. The patient is partially dependent on the respirator:

It is the most frequent case for severe CRI patients in whom a tracheostomy has been performed during the ICU period.

In most of those cases, the tracheostomy is maintained during a variable period after which there will be discussion as to whether to close it, or to keep it in order to install a long term home mechanical ventilation.

3. The patient has been completely weaned from the respirator:

Two possibilities are possible here:

3.1. If the patient has been tracheostomized during the acute episode, the question will be to close the tracheostomy before return home. The patient can easily leave the intensive care unit, and the decision to keep the tracheostomy or not is based upon the previous course of the disease responsible for CRI, and the tolerance of the interruption of the mechanical ventilation. Non-invasive mechanical ventilation by nasal/facial mask may be used with the most severe patients after the closure of the tracheostomy.

3.2. If the patient has not been tracheostomized, he can be quickly discharged from the ICU. It will be important to discuss the need for long-term oxygentherapy, specially for patients with COPD. It is well known, however, that it is necessary to wait some weeks or months[4] for some patients to decide the effective treatment at home, because their arterial blood gases may spontaneously improve after the ARF period.

Nowadays, in the most severe of those patients, when the respiratory status is unstable, a general trend is to rest the respiratory muscles using non-invasive devices as nasal or facial masks. Those techniques seem most effective in restrictive patients, especially in neuromuscular diseases.

Thus, dismission criteria from ICU are primarily governed in severe CRI patients by the control of the vital functions and their precipitating factors. The assessment of the respiratory function is then a long procedure which leads frequently to home ventilatory assistance.

It is the reason why specific units devoted to the preparation to long term ventilatory assistance, called "chronic ventilatory care units"[3] are required to provide to those patients and their relatives sociopsychological assistance as well as medical and technical education before going back home.

References

1. ACCP subcommittee of respiratory care section: Long-term mechanical ventilation: Guidelines for management in the home and at alternate community sites. Chest 1986; 90: 1(suppl.), 15-375
2. O'Ryan J.A. et al.: *Pulmonary rehabilitation: From hospital to home.* Year Book Medical Publishers, Inc., Vol. I 1984; 260
3. Calves P. et al.: An in-hospital chronic ventilatory unit positively affects patient outcome. Am. Rev. Respir. Dis. 1990; 141: 4, A572
4. G.E.M.O.S. (Multicentric study): Three months follow-up. Am. Rev. Respir. Dis. 1986; 133: 547-551

14. From Intensive Care to Home through Rehabilitation: Discharging Criteria For Patients on Partial Ventilatory Support

S. Zanaboni, S. Zaccaria, E. Zaccaria, L. Appendini, C.F. Donner

Division of Pulmonary Disease, Clinica del Lavoro Foundation, Institute of Care and Research, Medical Center of Rehabilitation, Veruno, Italy

Introduction

Intensive care unit (ICU) management of patients on partial ventilatory support is very expensive. To make this task cost effective, we opened a subintensive respiratory care unit (RCU) that is concerned with in-hospital and home care of patients who need mechanical ventilation for 8 hours a day at least. The procedure of discharging these patients to home is quite complex and requires multidisciplinary interventions. The clinical status is not the unique aspect to be evaluated before the hospital dismission of the patient. The following problems should also be faced: management; patient care, medical equipment; funding. In this paper we try to point out these major areas of concern.

The admission to an intensive care unit (ICU) can be lifesaving but can also create a ventilator dependent patient. Since hospital charges for ventilator-assisted patients are very expensive,[1] and ICU beds are relatively insufficient, ventilator dependent patients, also identified as "chronically critically ill patients",[2] need a less expensive structure that could take care of their management in and their discharge from the hospital to home or to alternative community sites. The goals of a "so called" subintensive respiratory care unit (RCU) are not exhausted in the hospital but extend to home care. Briefly, they are:

1. during hospitalization:
a. to save ICU beds for acute patients, receiving chronically critically ill patients from medical-ICU when they need ventilator support and medical care up to

class III patients according to TISS;[3]

b. to wean and improve the clinical conditions in order to discharge patients to a pulmonary division;
c. to evaluate the most useful therapy to prevent the worsening of clinical status;
2. after hospitalization:
a. to support severely ill patients by home mechanical ventilation (HMV).

It is to be stressed that patients admitted to subintensive respiratory care unit do not overlap with ICU patients. The former group is characterized by the following requirements:

1. to be in a chronic status of respiratory illness;
2. to need long term mechanical ventilation;
3. if completely ventilator dependent, to have some chance of being out of mechanical ventilation at least a few hours a day after weaning;
4. to have some perspective of improving the quality of life through rehabilitation programmes and long-term mechanical ventilation.

Successful applications of long-term partial ventilatory support have been performed in neuromuscular or restrictive diseases.[4-7] Its effectiveness in chronic obstructive pulmonary disease is still debated.[8,9] Whatever the primary home disease, ventilated patients need much more care than common patients, so discharging criteria must take into account not only clinical status, but also home care, management, medical equipment, and funding problems.

Clinical Status

Patients should have a relatively stable cardiopulmonary status, without wide fluctuations that require accurate monitoring and frequent readjustment of the therapy. Drugs should be orally administered in order to make home therapy and drug compliance easier. The type and daily duration of mechanical ventilation should be set and checked during an adequate period of time in which blood gases must range over safety limits. The connection to the respirator should be the least invasive according to the disease and the patient's clinical status. Usually, nasal/facial mask ventilation should be used in restrictive or neuromuscular diseases.[4-7] Up to now tracheostomy seems preferable in COPD patients even if there are some reports of successful treatment with the nasal mask.[10,11]

Supplemental oxygen should be titrated at this time with frequent arterial blood samples at different times during mechanical ventilation and spontaneous breathing. Arterial oxygen saturation should not be lower than 90% for at least 12-18 hours a day.[12,13]

A comprehensive respiratory function evaluation should be performed before discharging a patient from RCU, including respiratory mechanics with the measurement of airways pressure at 100 ms after the beginning of an occluded inspiratory effort (P0.1),[14] and of intrinsic positive end-expiratory pressure (PEEPi).[15] P0.1 represents an integrated index of inspiratory neuromuscular drive.[14]

Although its specificity can be questionable,[16] it seems to be a good weaning index from the ventilator.[17,18] In the context of the topic discussed in this paper, P0.1 may be an useful tool to assess the stability of clinical status[18] and to decide the more suitable treatment for the patient (weaning, HMV). Furthermore it can be helpful in the assessment of respiratory muscle fatigue.[18] During tidal breathing, the rate of lung emptying in COPD patients is impaired by increased pulmonary flow resistance and flow limitation; hence the end-expiratory lung volume is expected to be higher than the elastic equilibrium volume (or relaxation volume, Vr), a condition termed dynamic pulmonary hyperinflation (DH).[19-24]

DH is associated with the presence of a positive static end-expiratory elastic recoil pressure (Pst,rs), which has been called "auto PEEP"[25] or "intrinsic PEEP" (PEEPi).[21] PEEPi was demonstrated to compromise the inspiratory muscles while forcing them to operate against a greater elastic load and a threshold load,[26] and to be a determinant of ventilator dependence in chronic obstructive pulmonary disease (COPD).[19] Since PEEPi can be present also in stable COPD patients,[27] its monitoring can point out over time the load that respiratory muscles have to face, give a trend of respiratory mechanics impairment, and support therapeutic decisions taken on the basis of P0.1 measurements.

Management

The presence of a patient care coordinator is essential to assure the success of mechanical ventilation outside the hospital.[28] During the process of discharging patients, the coordinator has many responsibilities to face.

First, he has to supervise the discharge preparation evaluating the patient's status (see above), and to plan a comprehensive training program for the patient, his family, and caregivers (see below).

Second, he has to assess the suitability of the patient care outside the hospital. This task includes the evaluation of the care skills by the patient himself and caregivers, the inspection of the site for long term mechanical ventilation, the control of the proper operation of ventilator and other devices in the home environment, the finding of disposable supplies such as tracheostomy tubes and connectors, adaptors etc.

Third, he has to be a link between the patient, his family, physicians, ventilator service personnel, and all involved community-based health and personal care providers in order to make patient care and equipment maintenance more efficient.

Fourth, the determination of available reimbursement for patient care plan is a coordinator's duty too.

Fifth, he must supervise the initial transition from the hospital to home.

Patient Care

Patients, family, and caregivers should be trained for daily equipment maintenance and patient medical care. Before discharging the patient, all these subjects should be skilled in suctioning tracheal secretions, cleaning tracheostomy, changing cannulas (if tracheostomy is present), correctly positioning nasal mask and so on. This aim should be sought for with theoretical and practical sessions, written instructions, availability of equipment manuals covering all mechanical devices and accessories, audiovisual aids.

Patients, family, and caregivers should be instructed to face up to emergency in the eventuality of ventilator system malfunction. An emergency protocol should be provided for each ventilator-assisted patient transferred to the home.[28] Emergency procedures should be tailored to each patient according to the nature and severity of the respiratory disease, hours of dependence upon the ventilator each day, and physical functional capacity.

Some of these procedures have been recently stated:[28]
1. use of manual resuscitators;
2. use of emergency supplies;
3. phone numbers of emergency personnel (ambulance service, equipment vendors, physicians, and other home health personnel);
4. use of a backup mechanical ventilator.

We think that recognition and basic treatment of mechanical airways obstruction should also be taught.

Checking of the patient care skills acquired by the patient and caregivers is imperative, and responsibility for initial and ongoing teaching should be clearly defined.[28]

Medical Equipment

A list of needed equipment has been reported.[28] It is as follows:

1. Mechanical ventilator(s) and accessories, including backup power supply;
2. manual resuscitator and suction machine(s) for patients with a tracheostomy and others, as required;
3. ventilator and tracheostomy cleaning supplies;
4. oxygen equipment, as necessary;

5. ventilator and patient monitors and alarms, as prescribed by the physician;
6. communication, transportation, and assistance devices, as required.

Before discharging the patient to home, all these equipments must be acquired and patient and caregivers should be familiar with the respective operating procedures. The training should be performed initially in the hospital and then at home in order to avoid problems resulting from home installation (wrong AC connectors, inadequate number of sockets, incorrect power supply, too short oxygen tubings, etc.). In this phase, the testing of equipments will protect the patient against malfunctions due to factory faults.

Emergencies due to ventilator malfunction should be foreseen. If the patient is not routinely off the ventilator for 4 hours or more, or when a replacement ventilator cannot be provided within 2 hours, a backup ventilator will be necessary.[28]

Funding

HMV is costly even if it can prove cheaper than hospitalization of chronically ventilated patients.[29,30] A form of reimbursement should be found before discharging the patient to home. However, since several types of organization deal with HMV in different countries (state system in England, national insurance system in France, free market system in USA), it is impossible to give precise guidelines about this topic. Anyhow, reimbursement should be provided for the purchase of ventilator and other medical devices, for equipment surveillance, maintenance, and repair, and for medical and specialist assistance.[28] At present, reimbursement policy usually determines the number of patients who can benefit by HMV and its quality.[28,31,32]

For instance, in USA the Health Care Financing Administration (HCFA) added two new diagnosis related groups (DRG) in late 1987[33] in the attempt to reduce the difference between hospital costs and the paucity of reimbursement for patients requiring prolonged mechanical ventilation.

DRG 474 applied to patients receiving mechanical ventilation through a tracheostomy tube, and DRG 475 to similar patients receiving mechanical ventilation through an endotracheal tube. The weighting factors for DRGs 474 and 475 were 11.8772 and 3.1757, respectively. As a result of the great difference between the two factors, undue pressure was placed on physicians to perform tracheostomies prematurely.[31,32] Greater effort should be made to put in place the necessary reimbursement mechanisms to accomplish significantly improved quality of care and cost savings.

In conclusion, the dismission of a patient from RCU is a demanding task that requires multidisciplinary expertise and a lot of work in and outside the hospital. The result is the successful discharge of the patient assessed by extended life, the amelioration of quality of life, the enhancement of individual potential, the improvement of his physical and physiologic functions, and the increase of the cost/benefit ratio.

References

1. Wagner D.P.: Economics of prolonged mechanical ventilation. Am. Rev. Respir. Dis. 1989; 140: S14-S18
2. Raffin T.A.: Intensive care unit survival of patients with systemic illness. Am. Rev. Respir. Dis. 1989; 140: S28-S35
3. Keene A.R., Cullen D.J.: Therapeutic Intervention Scoring System: update 1983. Crit. Care Med. 1983; 11:1
4. Bach J.R., Alba A., Bohatiuk J., Saporito L., Lee M.: Mouth intermittent positive pressure ventilation in the management of postpolio respiratory insufficiency. Chest 1987; 91: 859-864
5. Kerby G.R., Mayer L.S., Pingleton S.K.: Nocturnal positive pressure ventilation via nasal mask. Am. Rev. Respir. Dis. 1987; 135: 738-740
6. Segall D.: Noninvasive nasal mask-assisted ventilation in respiratory failure of Duchenne muscular dystrophy. Chest 1988; 93:1298-1300
7. Bach J.R., Alba A., Mosher R., Delaubier A.: Intermittent positive ventilation via nasal access in the management of respiratory insufficiency. Chest 1987; 92:168-170
8. IPPB trial group. Intermittent positive pressure breathing therapy of chronic obstructive pulmonary disease. A clinical trial. Ann. Intern. Med. 1983; 99(5): 612-620
9. Branthwaite M.A.: Mechanical ventilation at home. Br. Med. J. 1989; 298: 1409
10. Brochard L., Isabey D., Piquet J., Amaro P., Mancebo J., Messadi A.A., Brun-Buisson C., Rauss A., Lemaire F., Harf A.: Reversal of acute exacerbations of chronic obstructive lung disease by inspiratory assistance with a face mask. N. Engl. J. Med. 1990; 323: 1523-1530
11. Carroll B., et al.: Non-invasive positive-pressure ventilation. In: *Proc. International Conference on Pulmonary Rehabilitation and Home Mechanical Ventilation,* Denver, 2-5 March, 1988 (Abstr.)
12. BMRC Working Party: Long-term domiciliary oxygentherapy in chronic hypoxic cor pulmonale complicating chronic bronchitis and emphysema. Lancet 1981; 1: 681-686
13. NOTT Group: Continuous or nocturnal oxygentherapy in hypoxaemic COPD. Ann. Intern. Med. 1980; 93: 391-398
14. Whitelaw W.A., Derenne J.P., Milic-Emili J.: Occlusion pressure as a measure of respiratory center output in conscious man. Respir. Physiol. 1975; 23: 181-199
15. Marini J.J.: Monitoring during mechanical ventilation. Clin. Chest Med. 1988; 9: 73-100
16. Marazzini L., Cavestri R., Gori D., Gatti L., Longhini E.: Difference between mouth and esophageal occlusion pressure during CO_2 rebreathing in chronic obstructive pulmonary disease. Am. Rev. Respir. Dis. 1978; 118: 1027-1033
17. Sassoon C.S.H., Te T.T., Mahutte C.K., Light R.W.: Airway occlusion pressure. An important indicator for successful weaning in patients with chronic obstructive pulmonary disease. Am. Rev. Respir. Dis. 1987; 135: 107113
18. Murciano D., Boczkowski J., Lecocguic Y., Milic-Emili J., Pariente R., Aubier M.: Tracheal occlusion pressure: a simple index to monitor respiratory muscle fatigue during acute respiratory failure in patients with chronic obstructive pulmonary disease. Ann. Intern. Med. 1988; 108(6): 800-805

19. Kimball W.R., Leith D.E., Robins A.G.: Dynamic hyperinflation and ventilator dependence in chronic obstructive pulmonary disease. Am. Rev. Respir. Dis. 1982; 126: 991-995

20. Gottfried S.B., Rossi A., Higgs B.D., et al.: Noninvasive determination of respiratory system mechanics during mechanical ventilation for acute respiratory failure. Am. Rev. Respir. Dis. 1985; 131: 414-420

21. Rossi A., Gottfried S.B., Zocchi L., et al.: Measurement of static compliance of the total respiratory system in patients with acute respiratory failure during mechanical ventilation. Am. Rev. Respir. Dis. 1985; 131: 672-677

22. Fleury B., Murciano D., Talamo C., Aubier M., Pariente R., Milic-Emili J.: Work of breathing in patients with chronic obstructive pulmonary disease in acute respiratory failure. Am. Rev. Respir. Dis. 1985; 131: 822-827

23. Gottfried S.B., Rossi A., Milic-Emili J.: Dynamic hyperinflation, intrinsic PEEP, and the mechanically ventilated patient. Intensive Crit. Care Digest 1986; 5: 30-33

24. Broseghini C., Brandolese R., Poggi R., et al.: Respiratory mechanics during the first day of mechanical ventilation in patients with pulmonary edema and chronic airway obstruction. Am. Rev. Respir. Dis. 1988; 138: 355-361

25. Pepe P.E., Marini J.J.: Occult positive end-expiratory pressure in mechanically ventilated patients with airflow obstruction. Am. Rev. Respir. Dis. 1982; 126: 166-170

26. Younes M.: Load responses, dyspnea, and respiratory failure. Chest 1990; 97(3) supplement: 59s-68s

27. Dal Vecchio L., Polese G., Poggi R., Rossi A.: "Intrinsic" positive end-expiratory pressure in stable patients with chronic obstructive pulmonary disease. Eur. Respir. J. 1990; 3(1): 74-80

28. Plummer A.L., O'Donohue W.J., Petty T.L.: Consensus conference on problems in home mechanical ventilation. Am. Rev. Respir. Dis. 1989; 140: 555-560

29. Haynes N., Raine S.F., Rushing P.: Discharging ICU ventilator-dependent patients to home healthcare. Crit. Care Nurse 1990; 10(7): 39-47

30. Fischer D.A.: Long-term management of the ventilator dependent patient: levels of disability and resocialization. Eur. Respir. J. 1989; 2(Suppl 7): 651-654

31. Plummer A.L., Gracey D.R.: Consensus conference on artificial airways in patients receiving mechanical ventilation. Chest 1989; 96(1): 178-180

32. Douglass P.S., Bone R.C., Rosen R.L.: DRG payment for long-term ventilator patients revisited. Chest 1988; 93(3): 629-631

33. Health Care Financing Agency. Federal Register 52FR 33143, Sep 1,1987

15. Home Care for Respiratory Patients: the Comprehensive Approach

N. DARDES, M.A. RE, L. PELLICCIOTTI, L. RUSSO, S. VULTERINI

Fatebenefratelli General Hospital, Isola Tiberina, Rome, Italy

Introduction

In the last ten years, clinical research in pneumology led to the important development whereby the long term application of a highly specialized therapy (such as mechanical ventilation or oxygen-therapy) determines a significant improvement in the survival of patients suffering from severe respiratory failure.[1,2] Consequently, the concept of home care took root in the culture of respiratory specialist.[1]

The concept of home care for respiratory disease, however, is still related exclusively to two elements:

1. Improvement of survival.
2. Application of specialized technology such as mechanical ventilation or oxygen, therapy.

Experience in other medical fields, such as oncology, geriatrics, nutrition or nephrology, shows that consideration of only these two elements offers an incomplete evaluation of results and inadequate efficacy of the home care programs.[1]

In fact, according to the specialists of basic medical sciences,[1,2] it is necessary to consider that the success of an exacting medical or surgical treatment cannot be evaluated merely in terms of survival, without taking into account another important parameter such as the quality of life.

The evaluation of quality of life is important not only to determine an overall judgement of the treatment's efficacy, but also to have the possibility of operating directly on it, adopting the necessary measures aimed at improving it.[3,4]

As to the second point it is necessary to underline that the home care of a patient, suffering from respiratory disease, does not involve exclusively problems related to mechanical ventilation or oxygen-therapy: it is also important to take into account other general medical problems.

In fact, being not prepared to manage at home other concomitant pathologies, such as diabetes mellitus, nutritional disorders, cardiovascular, urologic or orthopedic pathologies, can lead to the failure of treatment or, at least, to a significant reduction of its advantages.

Two other important elements have emerged either from experience in other medical fields or from the first experience of home care in respiratory pathology:[1,2]

1. the capacity of the home environment to receive the patient;
2. the training of caregivers.

Home Environment

The house in which the patient will be received must meet several requirements necessary for the success of the home care program. Such requirements are, of course, variable, depending on the pathology treated. The following home characteristics should be required for patients suffering from severe respiratory failure:

- *Care Space:* it is usually identified with a bedroom large enough for the necessary equipment (ventilator, oxygen tank, etc.) to be placed near the bed; a table for medicines and aerosol-therapy is required, as well as a space to perform the infusion therapy. A single bed is preferred to a double bed in order to make the physiotherapist's work possible.

- *Rehabilitation Space:* a covered space large enough to allow the exercise training would be possibly required in the flat, house or the immediate neighborhood. A course of a minimum of 25-30 months is necessary in order to allow the patient to train every day or more than once a day without feeling uncomfortable.
  If such spaces are not available in the house, it is possible to effect slight changes of the furnishings or of the wall structure, which, according to our experience, can be given consideration in flats larger than 100 m². Moreover rehabilitation spaces easily recoverable are represented by: cellars' or garages' corridors as well as by wash-spaces (widespread in central and southern Italy) situated on the top floor (provided that a lift is available). Last but not least, it will be necessary to make bathrooms more suitable to the patient's needs and also to eliminate architectural barriers such as stairs.

Caregivers

The staff's training plays an important role in the realization of home care. In fact, it is closely related to the optimization of management costs.[5] Two categories of staff should be employed in the realization of home care: professionals and non-professionals.

Professionals are represented by: physicians, rehabilitation therapists (respiratory and non-respiratory), nurses and general supporting personnel. In this group of professional, the physicians have exclusively a consultative and supervisory role. The others, on the contrary, play a more operative role, each according to his own competence, which, however, should be transferred, as much as possible, to the non-professional staff, trained by means of specific instruction programs. Consequently, therapists and nurses would also play simply a supervisory role, intervening only periodically.

The non-professional are represented, first of all, by the patient himself, who, depending on disease degree, education level and psychological status, can be employed in the care of himself.

Relatives and non-relatives, if present at home for a sufficient number of hours, can have the role of caregivers after adequate training. Support can also be given by other person such as neighbours, friends or household staff, who, however, would have a role of minor responsibility (in the absence of kin), that is general assistance, not strictly linked with the patient's care.

Generally housework can be easily done by friends or neighbors.

Involving relatives in the home care program presents numerous problems that go beyond the simple medical and nursing training, which can be quite easily acquired. In fact, it is necessary to take into account several elements, which make both patients and relatives accept or reject a care program.[7] These elements can be summarized as follows:

1. Quality of personal relationships before the onset of the disease.
2. Development of patient's dependence on his/her caregivers.
3. Patient's refusal of the dependence on a relative.
4. Duration of availability of the relative.
5. Availability of the relative to give his/her support also during weekends and holidays.
6. State of anxiety in recognizing and managing the first phases of possible emergency.
7. Stress, for having accepted the responsibility of care.

Therefore, the non-professionals' involvement in the home care can be carried out after the evaluation of the objective availability and family relationships.

The realization of Home Care in patients suffering from respiratory diseases foresees, therefore, the examination of numerous problems that determine the success of the program, in which several competences are required.

The International Home Care Association promoted a study on patients, suffering from chronic respiratory insufficiency, treated at home by the staff of Pneumology Unit - Hospital Fatebenefratelli General Hospital, Isola Tiberina, Rome.

The study was aimed at evaluating medical and organizational problems experienced during 1 year.

Patients and Methods

41 patients discharged after an episode of acute respiratory failure have been enrolled in the home care program and were followed up through one year. Age was on average 64±9 yrs; 35 subjects were males, 6 females.

Respiratory failure was related to COPD in 64% of cases, to Pulmonary Fibrosis in 5%, to Kyphoscoliosis in 3% and to other causes in 28%.

All patients were treated by Long Term Oxygen (LTD). Pharmacological therapy was given orally in most cases in a regimen ranging between two and ten tablets per day. Nebulizers for inhaled therapy were regularly used in 23 subjects (56%), and infusional therapy was very rare. The following items were evaluated in all cases:

1. Concomitant diseases.
2. Compliance to the treatment.
3. Recurrence of the respiratory symptoms in acute form.
4. Quality of life (Q.L.).
5. Environmental conditions.
6. Requirements for nursing care.

Quality of life was evaluated in all subjects by a questionnaire administered by a physician or by a trained technician on the occasion of a routine follow up visit. The questionnaire was aimed at evaluating the three main dimensions of Q.L. (e.g. Physical Well Being, Psychological Status and Social Activities). This method allows us to obtain a score expressing the extent of the impairment of Q.L.

Environmental conditions were judged by the staff as comfortable or not comfortable, taking into account the availability of the spaces for care or rehabilitation considering the possibility of carrying out modifications in the furnishings or minimal architectural changes.

According to the rules given by the Italian Health Ministery for the hospices, the minimum surface necessary for the care spaces was considered to be 9 m^2 (or 12 m^2 if another person is intended to sleep with the patient). From the practical point of view 3 m² of floor surface free from furnishings plus 1 m² for technology was considered the minimum requirement for the care space.

A short training program was carried out for the relatives or other non-professional caregivers and the requirements for nursing or medical care during the follow up were applied to evaluate the efficiency of the "non-professional care program".

Results

Concomitant diseases

12 out of 41 subjects were free from diseases other than respiratory failure requiring nursing or medical care. The management of diabetes mellitus was included in the Home Care Program in 12 subjects suffering from this disease.

Congestive heart failure was present in 5 cases, liver cirrhosis in 1 and hemiparesis in 1 patient. 4 subjects required management of urogenital disorders and 2 patients suffered from severe orthopedic diseases which required adequate treatment.

Compliance

The compliance to the medical regimen was good in 37 out of the 41 patients. 3 cases refused the medical treatment whereas one subject refused the rehabilitative program. The daily duration of oxygen-therapy judged by the average oxygen consumption was 14.4±2.3 hours per day.

Recurrence of acute respiratory symptoms

Acute episodes of dyspnea were very frequent (more than 2 episodes per week) in 11 subjects, asthma attacks requiring hospital admittance occurred in 8 cases, whereas 6 patients were admitted to hospital because of acute episodes of bronchitis followed by acute respiratory failure.

Quality of life

According to the standard obtained in our laboratory the ideal score for subjects aged between 65 and 75 years is 81. The average value obtained in our subjects was 37.8±10.4 whereas the score recorded in ambulatory patients suffering from chronic disease such as diabetes or cardiac failure was 56±12. The dimensions of quality of life mainly affected were Physical Well Being and Psychological Status whereas Social Relationships were almost normal.

148

Caregivers

As far as the Caregivers are concerned only 4 patients required the continuous intervention of professionals. Two subjects had no relatives able to take care of them. One subject had worsened familial relationship and one subject refused the intervention of non-professional caregivers.

The quality of care given by relatives (spouse 63%, sons 21%, others 7%) was judged satisfactory in all the 37 subjects. In fact the intervention of the staff or of the general pratictioner was required at weekly intervals in 12% of subjects, twice a month in 17% and at monthly intervals in 31%. In 39% of cases, the visits were less frequent than 1 visit per month.

Environmental Conditions

Judged confortable enough in 26 subjects and non-comfortable in the other 15 cases according to the criteria indicated above.

Conclusions

The present study has been carried out in order to evaluate the organizational problems emerging from a comprehensive approach to home care for severely disabled respiratory patients.

The results are not yet definitive and several problems need further investigation. Nonetheless some suggestions can be found in our data.

First of all, the need of a comprehensive medical approach seems to be mandatory, considering that more than 50% of patients enrolled in the home care program for respiratory failure have serious medical problems to be managed.

For this reason, even if the main problem requires the competence of respiratory specialists, the staff of the home care unit should be composed in a multidisciplinary way. According to our previous reports Quality of Life has significantly improved in patients suffering from severe respiratory failure, whereas the compliance to the treatment can be considered satisfactory probably due to the educational program. The approach to quality of life improvement is quite complex and unequivocal results are not yet reported in literature.

The non-comfortable environmental conditions represented a serious problem in many patients. The resolution of such problems probably requires organizational and economic efforts that will be considered in future planning.The employment of non-professional caregivers gave us satisfactory results, the refusal of the patient or of the relatives to participate in the care program being very rare.

Research carried out under the auspices of International Home Care Association, General Secretariat: 00136, Rome, Via Friggeri 55

References

1. Spitzer W.O.: State of sciences 1986: Quality of life and functional status as target variables for research. J. Chron. Dis. 1987; 40: 465-471
2. Katz S.: The science of quality of life. J. Chron. Dis. 1987; 40: 459-463
3. Dudley D.L., Glaser E.M., Jorgenson B.N., Logan D.L.: Psychosocial concomitants to rehabilitation in Chronic Obstructive Pulmonary Disease. Chest 1980; 77: 413-420
4. Prigatano G.P., Wright E.C., Levin D.: Quality of life and its predictors in patients with mild hypoxemia and chronic obstructive pulmonary disease. Arch. Intern. Med. 1984; 144: 1613-1619
5. Collopy B., Dubler N., Zuckerman C.: The ethics of Home Care: autonomy and accommodation. Hostin Center Reports: March-April 1990; 1-16
6. Brody E.M.: Parent care as a normative family stress. The Gerontologist 1985; 25: 19-29

16. Long Term Strategies for Respiratory Muscle Rest

N. AMBROSINO, C. FRACCHIA, C. RAMPULLA, R. CORSICO

Division of Pulmonary Disease, Clinica del Lavoro Foundation, Institute of Care and Research, Medical Center of Rehabilitation, Montescano, Pavia, Italy

Inspiratory muscle (IM) fatigue may be a cause of hypercapnic respiratory failure.[1] Muscle fatigue is defined as a condition in which there is a loss in the capacity for developing force and/or velocity in response to a load and which is reversible by rest.[2] IM may become fatigued in chronic diseases of airways (COPD), in restrictive lung and chest wall diseases (RTD) and in neuromuscular diseases (NMD). Ventilatory failure of patients with acute severe asthma or who fail to be weaned from mechanical ventilation (MV) may be the result of IM fatigue.[3] Regardless of the mechanism, the rest should be the best treatment of fatigued IM. The hypothesis that hypercapnia in stable COPD may be caused by a state of chronic muscle fatigue has been questioned, so that according to the afore-mentioned definition of fatigue, benefits arising from IM rest, if any, might be considered as a demonstration *ex juvantibus* of the existence of chronic IM fatigue. This situation is however not easy to be proven due to the fact that IM rest is usually delivered by means of MV, so that it is not easy to know whether benefits depend on rest or ventilatory effects or both.

Inclusion Criteria

Several criteria have been proposed to be predictive of the need of IM rest by MV.[4]

Clinical Criterial

Severe, irreversible disease; frequent relapses of the disease; deterioration after successful weaning; sleep disturbances; severe dyspnea; increasing tachypnea; paradox or asynchrony; cor pulmonale despite conventional treatment.

Pulmonary Function Criteria

VC   < 25% predicted
FEV_1 < 25% predicted
MVV < 25% predicted
MIP   < 50 cm H_2O in COPD and TRD
       < 25 cm H_2O in NMD
MEP > 40 cm H_2O
$PaCO_2$ > 45 mmHg

No single criterion can be an absolute indication for IM rest but several together make it more likely to be necessary. Efforts should be made to determine clinical and physiological scores in indications for IM rest.

Goals of IM Rest

The final goals for IM rest should be to preserve or increase the capacity for daily living and to prevent deterioration of function. Survival cannot be considered as an absolute criterion of successful therapy.

Preliminary Evaluation

To be included in programs of IM rest patients should undergo a detailed history and physical examination, an evaluation of nutritional status and a psychosocial profile for a better prognosis for compliance. Only highly motivated patients can get advantage from this kind of treatment.[5] The more depressed the patient and the greater the degree of psychological problems before the institution of a system, the less likely the success of treatment. Psychological sets predictive for compliance to treatment should be determined.

Physiological Assessment and Monitoring

1. Pulmonary function.
2. Blood gases.
3. Respiratory muscle strength and endurance.
4. Cardiac function.
5. Sleep studies.
6. Electromyographic studies.

While these assessments are being made, patients must undergo maximal drug therapy and comprehensive respiratory rehabilitation programs including chest physical therapy to clear airways, relaxation and energy conservation techniques. Patients, family members and caregivers should be educated about the disease and on the use of devices to be prescribed. It is best to institute a system in the hospital where the questions, fear and panic of the patient can be addressed by the professional staff and the patient's physician.

On the other hand institution of a system at home rather than in the hospital reduces costs,[6] and may avoid the risk of nosocomial infections. Symptomatic demonstration of the usefulness of the devices is the best incentive to their use by patients. The simplest device to fit our purposes is the one to be selected. Several models may have to be tried until the most suitable one is found for the patient and the family.[7]

The main preliminary evaluation to be performed is the ventilatory set, if any, able to provide real IM rest. It may be not practical to invasively determine indices of IM activity in the routine clinical setting, but recording of diaphragm electromyographic activity from surface electrodes is a simple noninvasive method which can be used to ensure that IM are being effectively rested. Much trial and error may be necessary before the appropriate ventilatory set and patient's familiarization with the device afford a real IM rest. The observation during MV of a 50% reduction of electromyographic activity in the diaphragm as assessed by surface electrodes, in comparison to spontaneous breathing, should be considered as an index of IM rest.

Devices for Long Term IM Rest

Technical description of these devices has widely been reported by Hill.[8]

Diaphgram Movers

Rocking bed. It uses gravity to passively move the diaphragm via the abdominal contents. Tidal volumes are not controlled and IM rest is not achieved by this device.[9] It has been used in the treatment of severely paretic or paralyzed diaphragm, expecially in phrenic nerve damage due to cardiac by-pass surgery.[10, 11] *Pneumobelt.* This device enhances exhalation forcing the diaphragm up. Tidal volumes are not easily controlled and are influenced by the patient's size. It is used in diaphragmatic paralysis and it cannot be considered as a device to rest respiratory muscles.

Intermittent Negative Pressure Ventilators

IM can be unloaded in COPD patients by the application of cyclic negative pressure to the chest wall[12] by iron lung or cuirass and poncho wrap ventilators. Confirming previous work more recent reports indicate that intermittent negative pressure ventilation (INPV) performed by these devices is able to rest IM after a period of adaptation,[9, 12-15] although Rodenstein et al. considered these changes as influenced by behavioral factors[16, 17] and Henke et al. showed that positive pressure ventilation was more effective in eliminating phasic respiratory activity than was INPV, at least in the first few minutes.[18]

INPV has been considered an effective method of preventing sleep-induced reductions in alveolar ventilation and a practical method of long term management of patients with NMD and TRD.[19]

Side Effects of INPV

Ventilation with positive pressures was found to affect venous return and cardiac output.[20] Iron lung has been shown to affect venous return[21] while no adverse hemodynamic effect has been observed during cuirass ventilation in COPD patients.[22]

During INPV by poncho wrap ventilators some patients develop airway occlusion so this kind of ventilation is not be prescribed during sleep if specific sleep studies under INPV have not been performed.[23]

Schedule of Treatment

The possible therapeutic value of daily INPV was signaled by Braun and Marino[24] who reported significant improvements in IM strength, blood gases, and VC in 18 COPD patients who received ventilation for 4-10 hours/day for several months.

Shorter applications (3 to 6 hours/day per 3 to 5 consecutive days) of IM rest showed significant short term improvements in patients with severe COPD and respiratory failure,[14, 25] the benefits lasting no longer than 5 days.

Gutierrez et al. found in an uncontrolled study that an 8 hours once a week schedule with INPV in patients with respiratory failure was effective in long term treatment.[26] In contrast Zibrak et al., using a cross over design, failed to show any improvement in 20 patients with stable severe COPD encouraged to use INPV for 6 to 8 hours each day and to try to sleep overnight using the ventilator. 11 of the patients were unable to tolerate ventilator treatment, and the compliance with treatment was limited (average of INPV: 4.1 hours/day). The degree of IM rest was not objectively assessed.[27] Celli et al. rested IM as assessed clinically and/or by electromyography encouraging patients to use ventilators as many hours as tolerated. On a daily basis most patients chose to use ventilators 4.5 hours/day in the late evening and early night. This schedule did not result in increased benefit over that achieved by a comprehensive pulmonary rehabilitation program although the one patient with the highest $PaCO_2$ significantly improved.[28]

Montreal randomized double blind placebo controlled clinical trial of home INPV in 184 COPD patients randomized to sham or active INPV for 8 hours/day did not show effectiveness of active INPV versus sham treatment observed during training active INPV trial in each patient.[29]

In conclusion, to date much more study is needed to determine the optimal times for IM rest by INPV. Demonstration of effective IM rest by electromyographic studies should be mandatory before beginning long term treatment with INPV.

Intermittent Positive Pressure Ventilation by Nasal Route

Non invasive intermittent positive pressure ventilation applied through a nasal mask (NIPPV) has been shown to be useful in the treatment of chronic respiratory failure resulting from NMD, TRD and COPD.[30-33] It is usually delivered by standard volume cycled ventilators in assisted /control mode. Long term use of NIPPV has resulted in improvement in clinical status and in parameters of ventilatory function between treatments. NIPPV delivered in control mode has resulted in reductions of phasic diaphragmatic activity as assessed by a reduction in diaphragmatic electromyogram and by positive intrathoracic pressure swings on inspiration. Also a reduction in activity of accessory respiratory muscles has been observed.[34] Assisted mode of ventilation does not seem to be effective in resting IM.[35]

Side Effects

Reports describing the long term use of NIPPV have reported minimal side effects such as nasal abrasion,[31, 33] mask leaks[31] and abdominal distension,[33] none of which required discontinuation of NIPPV.

Schedule of Treatment

In order to provide maximum reduction of IM activity the ventilator settings must be individualized for each subject. NIPPV avoids upper airways obstruction and may be prescribed for nocturnal use. Demonstration of clinical usefulness should indicate the individual therapeutical schedule.

Choice of the Device

Selection of a device depends on the ability of the patient to cope with it, individual tolerance, availability of the device and financial resources of the patient. It is also important that physician and team become familiar with only a few devices . It seems that INPV can be applied effectively to NMD patients, while its application in COPD is limited to selected patients (mainly hypercapnic). NIPPV

156

seems promising not only in delivering MV but also in resting IM in all kind of patients. Other devices are not considered able to effectively rest IM.

Selection of Treatment Schedule

No optimal daytime duration of IM rest has been determined up to now. Out of an in-hospital setting patients may have the tendency to reduce ventilator time especially when they feel better. Further studies are necessary to determine the minimal effective daytime duration of treatment. No data indicate that respiratory muscles atrophy with rest induced by intermittent MV.

In fact both INPV and NIPPV have been shown to be able to reduce but not to continuously abolish IM activity. About half of the patients need to increase ventilatory support time, the NMD patients progressing to whole day ventilation more quickly than COPD and TRD patients.

References

1. Roussos C., Macklem P.T.: Diaphragmatic fatigue in man. J. Appl. Physiol. 1977; 43: 189-197
2. NHBLI Workshop: Respiratory muscle fatigue: report of the respiratory muscle fatigue workshop group. Am. Rev. Respir. Dis. 1990; 142: 474-480
3. Cohen C.A., Zagelbaum G., Gross D., Roussos C., Macklem P.T.: Clinical manifestations of inspiratory muscle fatigue. Am. J. Med. 1982; 73: 308-316
4. Rochester D.F., Martin L.L.: Respiratory muscle rest. In Roussos C., Macklem P.T. (Eds): *The Thorax*, part B. New York, Marcel Dekker, 1985, 1303-1328
5. Johnson D., Giovonni R.M., Discoll S.A.: *Ventilator assisted patient care. Planning for hospital discharge and home care*. Rockville MD, Aspen Pub., 1986, 1-23, 153-184.
6. AAR Times 1984; 28-31
7. Braun N.M.T.: Intermittent mechanical ventilation. Clinics in Chest Med. 1988; 9: 153-162
8. Hill N.S.: Clinical application of body ventilators. Chest 1986; 90: 897-905
9. Goldstein R.S., Molotiu N., Skrastins R., Long S., Contreras M.: Assisting ventilation in respiratory failure by negative pressure ventilation and by rocking bed. Chest 1987; 92: 470-474
10. Braun N.M.T., Faulkner J., Hughes R.L., Roussos C., Sahgal V.: When should respiratory muscle be exercised? Chest 1983; 84: 76-84
11. Abd A.G., Braun N.M.T., Baskin M.I., O'Sullivan M.M., Alkaitis D.A.: Diaphragmatic dysfunction after open heart surgery: treatment with a rocking bed. Ann. Intern. Med. 1989; 111: 881-886
12. Rochester D.F., Braun N.M.T., Laine S.: Diaphragmatic energy expenditure in chronic respiratory failure: the effect of assisted ventilation with body respirators. Am. J. Med. 1977; 63: 223-232
13. Scano G., Gigliotti F., Duranti R., Spinelli A., Gorini M., Schiavina M.: Changes in ventilatory muscle function with negative pressure ventilation in patients with severe COPD. Chest 1990; 97: 322-327
14. Ambrosino N., Montagna T., Nava S., Negri A., Brega S., Fracchia C., Zocchi L., Rampulla C.: Short term effect of intermittent negative pressure ventilation in COPD patients with respiratory failure. Eur. Respir. J. 1990; 3: 502-508

15. Nava S., Ambrosino N., Zocchi L., Rampulla C.: Diaphragmatic rest during negative pressure ventilation by pneumowrap. Assessment in normal and COPD patients. Chest 1990; 98: 857-865
16. Rodenstein D.O., Cutitta G., Stanescu D.C.: Ventilatory and diaphragmatic EMG changes during negative pressure ventilation in healthy subjects. J. Appl. Physiol. 1988; 64: 2272-2278
17. Rodenstein D.O., Stanescu D.C., Cutitta G., Liistro G., Veriter C.: Ventilatory and diaphragmatic EMG responses to negative pressure ventilation in airflow obstruction. J. Appl. Physiol. 1988; 65: 1621-1626
18. Henke K.G., Arias A., Skatrud J.B., Dempsey J.A.: Inhibition of inspiratory muscle activity during sleep. Chemical and non chemical influences. Am. Rev. Respir. Dis. 1988; 138: 8-15
19. Goldstein R.S., Molotiu N., Skrastins R., Long S., De Rosie J., Contreras M., Popkin J., Rutheford R., Phillipson E.A.: Reversal of sleep-induced hypoventilation and chronic respiratory failure by nocturnal negative pressure ventilation in patients with restrictive ventilatory impairment. Am. Rev. Respir. Dis. 1987; 1049-1056
20. Cournand A., Motley H.L., Werko L., Richards D.W. Jr: Physiological studies of the effects of intermittent positive pressure breathing on cardiac output in man. Am. J. Physiol. 1948; 23: 944-953
21. Beck G.J., Seanor H.E., Barach A.L., Gates D.: Effects of pressure breathing on venous pressure: a comparative study of positive pressure applied to the upper respiratory passageway and negative pressure to the body of normal individuals. Am. J. Med. Sci. 1952; 224: 169-174
22. Ambrosino N., Cobelli F., Torbicki A., Opasich C., Pozzoli M., Fracchia C., Rampulla C.: Hemodynamic effects of negative pressure ventilation in patients with COPD. Chest 1990; 97: 850-856
23. Levy R.D., Bradley T.D., Newman S.L., Macklem P.T., Martin J.G.: Negative pressure ventilation. Effects on ventilation during sleep in normal subjects. Chest 1989; 95: 95-99
24. Braun N., Marino W.D.: Effect of daily intermittent rest of respiratory muscles in patients with severe chronic airflow limitation. Chest 1984; 85: 595S
25. Cropp A., Di Marco A.F.: Effects of intermittent negative pressure ventilation in respiratory muscle function in patients with severe chronic obstructive pulmonary disease. Am. Rev. Respir. Dis. 1987; 135: 1056-1061
26. Gutierrez M., Beroiza T., Contreras G., Diaj O., Cruy E., Moreno R.R., Lisboa C.: Weekly cuirass ventilation improves blood gases and inspiratory muscle strength in patients with chronic air-flow limitation and hypercarbia. Am. Rev. Respir. Dis. 1988; 136: 617-623
27. Zibrak J.D., Hill N.S., Federman E.C., Kwa S.L., O'Donnell C.: Evaluation of intermittent long-term negative pressure ventilation in patients with severe chronic obstructive pulmonary disease. Am. Rev. Respir. Dis. 1988; 138: 1515-1518
28. Celli B., Lee H., Criner G., Bermudez M., Rassulo J., Gilmartin M., Miller G., Make B.: Controlled trial of external negative pressure ventilation in patients with severe chronic airflow obstruction. Am. Rev. Respir. Dis. 1989; 140:1251-1256
29. Martin J.G. : Clinical intervention in chronic respiratory failure. Chest 1990; 97 (Supplement): 105S-109S
30. Ellis E.R., Bye P.T.P., Bruderer J.W., Sullivan C.E.: Treatment of respiratory failure during sleep in patients with neuromuscular disease: positive-pressure ventilation through a nose mask. Am. Rev. Respir. Dis. 1987; 135: 148-152
31. Kerby G.R., Mayer L.S., Pingleton S.K.: Nocturnal positive pressure ventilation via nasal mask. Am. Rev. Respir. Dis. 1987; 135: 738-740
32. Bach J.R., Alba A., Mosher R., Delaubier A.: Intermittent positive pressure ventilation via nasal access in the management of respiratory insufficiency. Chest 1987; 92: 168-170
33. Carroll N., Branthwaite M.A.: Control of nocturnal hypoventilation by nasal positive pressure

ventilation. Thorax 1988; 43: 349-353

34. Carrey Z., Gottfried S.B., Levy R.D.: Ventilatory muscle support in respiratory failure with nasal positive pressure ventilation. Chest 1990; 97: 150-158

35. Marini J.J., Rodriguez R.M., Lamb V.: The inspiratory workload of patient initiated mechanical ventilation. Am. Rev. Respir. Dis. 1986; 134: 902-909

17. Heart Transplantation: Gas Exchange and Cardiovascular Readjustments

P. Cerretelli[1], M. Meyer[4], B. Grassi[3], M. Rieu[2], C. Cabrol[5], C. Marconi[3]

1.Physiology Laboratories, University of Geneva, Switzerland
2. Physiology Laboratories of Paris V, France
3. ITBA-CNR, Milan, Italy
4. Max Planck Institute Exp. Med., Göttingen, Germany
5. Department of Cardiovascular Surgery, Paris VI, France

Introduction

In slightly over two decades, cardiac transplantation has become an established treatment for end-stage heart disease. More recently, developments in combined heart-lung and lung transplantation techniques have also taken place. So far, as of October 1989, the Registry of the International Society for Heart Transplantation has collected data on some 11,000 heart transplant recipients (HTR), 591 heart-lung transplant recipients (HLTR) and 111 single/double lung transplant recipients.[1] The improved donor organ preservation and a more careful donor selection, along with new immunosuppressive treatment protocols, have improved the survival rate of both HTR and HLTR, thus prompting a number of physiological studies aimed at evaluating the functional conditions of these patients after surgery.

In this context, over the last three years, our group has performed a series of measurements on a total of 34 HTR and 4 HLTR.

The investigations were carried out on patients from the Centro De Gasperis, Niguarda Hospital, Milan, the Department of Cardiovascular Surgery of La Pitié-Salpétrière Hospital, Paris, and the Hôpital Cantonal Universitaire of Geneva. The present report includes, together with an outline of the techniques utilized, an analysis of:

a. the gas exchange in the lungs at rest and during exercise;

b. the cardiovascular readjustments occurring during steady-state graded exercise and during the rest-to-work transition;

c. the characteristics and the functional implications of the so-called metabolic or "lactic" anaerobic threshold.

Methods

Gas exchange measurements

Continuous monitoring on a breath-by-breath basis of pulmonary ventilation ($\dot{V}_E$), oxygen consumption ($\dot{V}O_2$), carbon dioxide output ($\dot{V}CO_2$), gas exchange ratio (RQ), and end-tidal O_2 and CO_2 partial pressures ($PETO_2$ and $PETCO_2$) was performed by a SensorMedics 4400tc analyzer. Tidal volume and ventilation were calculated integrating instantaneous flow tracings recorded at the mouth of the subject by a low-resistance turbine-flowmeter. Metabolic variables were determined by continuously monitoring PO_2 and PCO_2 throughout the respiratory cycle and from established mass balance equations.

The ventilation and gas exchange kinetics during the rest to work transients were calculated as half-time (t ^{1}/2, s) of the $\dot{V}_E$, $\dot{V}O_2$, and $\dot{V}CO_2$ on- and off-response curves, at the onset and offset, respectively, of imposed work loads, i.e. the time required to reach 50% of either the asymptotic (or peak) level starting from rest or, during the recovery, the resting value starting from the asymptotic level. Breath-by-breath recordings of $\dot{V}_E$, $\dot{V}O_2$ and $\dot{V}CO_2$ of a typical HTR at rest, during a constant-load (50 W) exercise and in the following recovery phase are shown in figure 1.

Monitoring of cardiovascular parameters

Beat-by-beat absolute stroke volume (SV) values as well as changes of cardiac output (Q) were recorded non-invasively by impedance cardiography. Cardiograms were obtained by means of an impedance device designed at the Department of Biomedical Engineering, University of Stuttgart. A constant current of 4 mA at a frequency of 100 kHz was introduced by two disposable self-adhesive electrodes.

Two separate electrodes were used to measure changes of voltage resulting from variations in impedance within the segment under consideration. The four-spot electrode array was placed according to Kubicek's scheme[2] with two electrodes 3 cm apart at the neck, the third at the level of the xiphisternal joint, and the fourth 3 cm below the third.

Baseline thoracic impedance (Z_0), changes of impedance (dZ/dt) and maximum of impedance derivative (dZ/dt max) were automatically derived along with estimates of pre-ejection period, left ventricular ejection time (LVET) and heart rate (HR). The stroke volume of the heart (SV) is calculated according to the formula of Kubicek et al.[2] knowing the distance (L) between the inner electrodes and the resistivity (ρ) of the blood at 100 kHz:

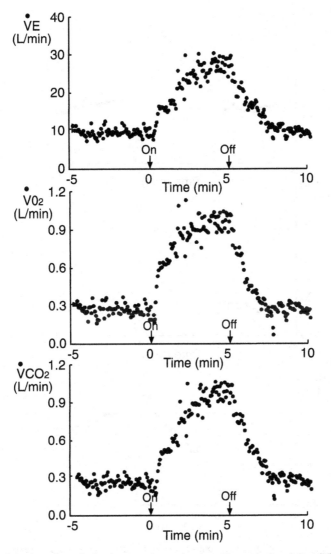

Fig. 1. Breath-by-breath analysis of gas exchange in a heart transplant recipient (HTR) at rest, during a constant-load 50 W cycloergometric exercise and in the following recovery.

$$SV = \rho \ (L/Z_0)^2 \ (dZ/dt_{max}) \ LVET$$

Continuous recordings of Q, SV and HR in a HTR while carrying out the same exercise protocol as adopted for assessing gas exchange (Fig.l) are shown in figure 2. The rate of readjustment ($t^{1/2}$) of Q upon the onset and offset of a constant load (50 W) exercise was evaluated as described previously for gas exchange.

162

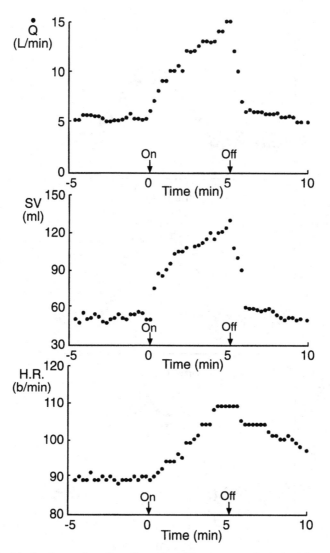

Fig. 2. Beat-by-beat recording of cardiac output (Q, upper panel), stroke volume (SV, middle panel) and heart rate (HR, lower panel) by impedance cardiography in a HTR at rest, during a constant-load 50 W cycloergometric exercise and in the following recovery.

Blood lactate and catecholamines concentration

Blood samples (20 µl) were taken from a pre-heated ear lobe. Blood lactate concentration [La$_b$] was determined by a lactate electrode (Kontron 640 Lactate Analyzer). In 10 HTR, blood samples were also taken from an indwelling jugular vein catheter (inserted for routine endomyocardial biopsy) for the analysis of both lactate and catecholamines. Plasma epinephrine (E) and norepinephrine (NE) were assessed by high pressure liquid chromatography (C-18 column) connected with an electrochemical detector (E.S.A. Coulom 5100 A).[3]

Results

A. Respiratory and metabolic variables
A1. Submaximal and maximal $\dot{V}O_2$ levels

As may be seen from figure 3, peak $\dot{V}O_2$ data of 17 HTR performing individual maximal cycloergometric tests (closed circles) are scattered over a wide range from 0.74 to 1.98 l/min. The average peak $\dot{V}O_2$ value is 1.30 ± 0.37 l/min (not shown in the figure). Shown in the same graph are also submaximal $\dot{V}O_2$ individual values for HTR (open circles), and average values for a group of 34 HTR (open squares) and for a group of 4 HLTR (triangles).

Both submaximal and maximal $\dot{V}O_2$ data for the investigated patients (HTR and HLTR) appear to cluster around the reference line for normal control subjects (CTL). This finding indicates that, despite the pharmacological treatment (prednisone, cyclosporine A, etc.), the mechanical efficiency of exercise was unchanged in the patients.

In analyzing the results of figure 3, it should be considered that some of the data, particularly those at higher work loads (>75 W), may underestimate the actual total energy requirement of the subjects, which, in fact, may also include ATP resynthetized by way of anaerobic glycolysis (see paragraph C).

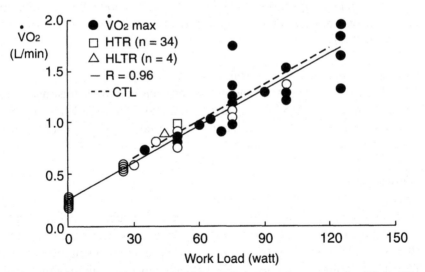

Fig. 3. Submaximal (open circles) and maximal (closed circles) oxygen consumption (VO_2) in 17 heart transplant recipients (HTR). (open squares) is the mean value of 34 HTR; (triangles) is the mean value of 4 heart-lung transplant recipients. Dashed line is the reference line for CTL.

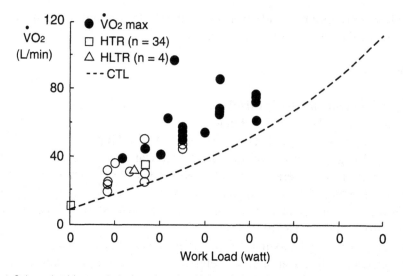

Fig. 4. Submaximal (open circles) and maximal (closed circles) pulmonary ventilation (VE) in 17 HTR. (open square) is the mean value of 34 HTR; (triangles) is the mean value of 4 heart-lung transplant recipients. Dashed line is the reference line for CTL.

A2. Submaximal and maximal ventilation

As shown in figure 4, the maximal pulmonary ventilation appears to be definitely lower ($\sim$ 80 l/min) in HTR than in normal sedentary CTL ($\sim$ 120 l/min). Moreover, mainly due to an enhanced respiratory rate both at rest or at any investigated work load, steady-state VE appears to be higher in both HTR and HLTR patients than in CTL. As a consequence, $PETCO_2$ is significantly lower than the corresponding value for the CTL.

A3. Gas exchange during the rest to work transient

The $t^{1/2}$ of the gas exchange and pulmonary ventilation readjustment upon the onset of a constant-load (50 W) cycloergometric exercise (Fig.1) are significantly longer in HTR than in CTL. Average (n=34) $t^{1/2}$ values of the $\dot{V}E, \dot{V}O_2$ and $\dot{V}CO_2$ on-responses are shown in figure 5.

B. Cardiovascular variables
B1. Heart rate

The HR values at rest and during steady-state (O_2) submaximal and peak work loads are those characteristic for chronically denervated hearts (i.e. those imposed by the "intrinsic" rate of the sinoatrial node). The average resting HR value on 21 HTR is 102±12 b/min. The average HR values at any given submaximal work load are essentially higher than the homologous (i.e. at the same absolute $\dot{V}O_2$) CTL values. Mean peak HR is 136 b/min (the highest measured HR was 154 b/min).

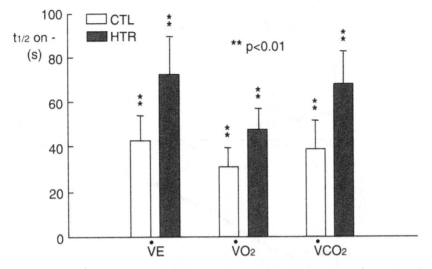

Fig. 5. Half-times (t¹/2 on-) of the VE, VO_2 and VCO_2 on-responses at the onset of a constant-load (50 W) exercise in HTR (filled bar) and in CTL (open bar).

HTR do not exhibit the usual age-dependent reduction of peak HR.[4] During the first minute of a constant-load exercise HR does not change, independent of the work load. HR increases thereafter almost linearly at a rate that is greater the heavier the load (Fig. 6). At the offset of exercise, HR after leveling off, or even further increasing (1-2 min) after the heaviest work loads, resume preexercise levels within 5-25 min, depending on the work load. The changes of HR appear to be related mainly, even though not exclusively,[5] to the level of circulating catecholamines.

B2. Catecholamines

Normal subjects are known to exhibit increased catecholamine levels during exercise. Similarly, a substantial increase of plasma norepinephrine has been observed by radio-enzymatic assay in HTR during severe exercise.[6] Moreover, it has been demonstrated recently that the denervated human heart exhibits adrenergic presynaptic supersensitivity of the sinus node to agents that are ordinarily removed by the neuronal uptake system.[7] Plasma catecholamine concentrations determined in 10 HTR (closed symbols) at rest and at different times (1,3,5 min) during a constant-load (50 W) cycloergometric exercise are shown as a function of HR in figure 7. Individual data collected at steady state on 2 HTR[4] are also shown.

The average resting plasma norepinephrine level collected while the patients were standing on the bike is nearly 850 pg/ml, i.e. 3-4 times higher than expected, thus indicating that a "true resting" condition was not achieved.

The role of catecholamines in the control of HR is demonstrated by the close relationship between norepinephrine levels and HR.

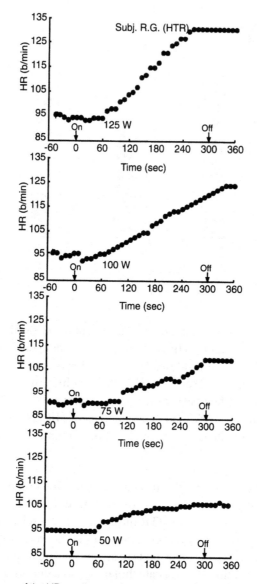

Fig. 6. Time course of the HR readjustment rate at the onset and offset of increasing rectangular work loads in a typical HTR.[4]

B3. Cardiac output

Cardiac output ($\dot{Q}$) at rest is essentially the same in HTR and in CTL (7.2±2.4 vs 6.8±1.5 l/min). Since HR in HTR is higher, the stroke volume (SV) is reduced compared to CTL (on the average 70 vs. 95 ml). During submaximal constant-load exercise (50W), steady-state $\dot{Q}$ is about 20% higher in HTR than in CTL (15.6 *vs*

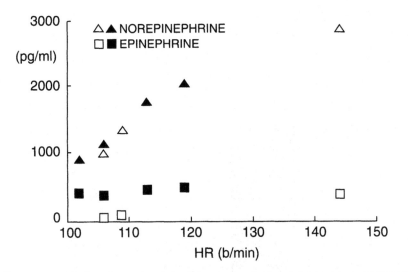

Fig. 7. Plasma concentration of norepinephrine (triangles) and epinephrine (open squares) in 10 HTR at rest and at 1,3,5 min of a constant-load (50 W) cycloergometric exercise as a function of HR. Individual data obtained in 2 HTR (open symbols) are also shown.[4]

12.8 l/min), whereas SV is practically the same (130 vs. 137 ml). Upon the onset of a constant-load (50 W) cycloergometric exercise, the kinetics of readjustment of $\dot{Q}$ appears to be only moderately reduced (52 ± 16 vs 40 ± 17 s, p>0.005) (Fig. 8). In HTR, in the absence of a normal fast HR readjustment, the rapid increase of $\dot{Q}$ at the onset of exercise reflects the nearly instantaneous increase of SV (Fig. 2), as a result of augmented venous return and the Frank-Starling mechanism.

C. Blood lactate and anaerobic threshold

Blood lactate concentration $[La_b]$ following voluntary exhaustion varies over a wide range, from 3.4 to 10.3 mM, as a consequence of the varying individual fitness level. During the rest to work transition, the rate of accumulation of La in blood ("early lactate") in HTR is not greatly different from that of CTL.[4]

Moreover, in spite of the well known muscle ultrastructural abnormalities due to prednisone administration,[8] the anaerobic threshold (AT) occurs at about the same percentage of $\dot{V}O_2max$ (50%) as in untrained CTL performing the same exercise protocol.

Conclusions

The present results indicate that chronically heart denervated human subjects (HTR and to a lesser extent HLTR) may develop compensatory reactions that are

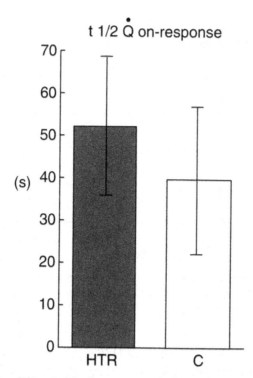

t 1/2 Q̇ on-response

(s)

HTR   C

Fig. 8. Half-time (tl/2 on-) of the Q on-response in the same condition as in Fig.5.

adequate to assure acceptable performances, from the standpoint of muscle energetics. In fact:

1. The maximal aerobic power may reach in HTR and in HLTR 60% and 40%, respectively, of that of CTL, i.e. 6-4 times respectively the resting level.
2. The efficiency of muscle contraction as determined from the $\Delta \dot{V}O_2/\Delta W$ ratio is essentially normal.
3. The catecholamine response to exercise for the same relative $\dot{V}O_2$ appears to be normal, and represents the major determinant of the readjustment of HR.
4. The increased stroke volume (SV) of the heart as a consequence of an enhanced Frank-Starling mechanism compensates for the lack of the HR response at the onset of exercise.
5. The rate of readjustment of the pulmonary gas exchange during the rest to work transition, particularly in HTR, is not reduced, in spite of the changes in the kinetics of cardiovascular readjustment.
6. The energy yield by anaerobic glycolysis is not affected by the immunosuppressive therapy.

The above conclusions are drawn from the results obtained in patients carrying out physical activities either professionally or for leisure out of programmed rehabilitation schemes. It is likely that specifically designed rehabilitation protocols may further improve their maximal muscular power and therefore their working capability.

Acknowledgement

The authors are grateful to all the patients who willingly collaborated in this study. The authors are also in debt to Mr. A. Colombini, Mr. M. Pellegrini and Miss L. Raimondi for their helpful assistance.
This work was supported by C.N.R. Special Target Biotechnology and Bioinstrumentation and Grant. 3.088-0.87 of the National Swiss Fonds for Scientific Research.

References

1. Kriett J.M., Tarazi R.Y., Kaye M.P.: The Registry of the International Society for Heart Transplantation. In: P. Terasaki (Ed.) *Clinical Transplants.* Los Angeles, California, UCLA Tissue Typing Laboratory, 1989; 45-53
2. Kubicek W.G., Karnegis J.M., Patterson R.P., Witsoe D.A., Mattson R.H.: Development and evaluation of an impedance cardiac output system. Aerosp. Med. 1966; 37:1208-1212
3. Mefford I.N., Ward M.M., Miles L., Taylor B., Chesney M.A., Keegan D.L., Barchas J.D.: Determination of plasma catecholamines and free 3,4-dihydroxyphenylacetic acid in continuously collected human plasma by high performance liquid chromatography with electrochemical detection. In: K. Brendel (Ed.) *Life Science.* London, Pergamon Press, 1981; vol 28, 477-588.
4. Cerretelli P., Grassi B., Colombini A., Caru' B., Marconi C.: Gas exchange and metabolic transients in heart transplant recipients. Respir. Physiol. 1988;74:355-371
5. Meyer M., Cerretelli P., Marconi C., Rieu M., Cabrol C.H.: Cardiorespiratory adjustment to exercise after cardiac transplantation. In: K. Reinhart and K. Eyrich (Eds.) *Clinical Aspects of O₂ Transport and Tissue Oxygenation.* Berlin, Springer-Verlag, 1989, 477-499
6. Pope S.E., Stinson E.B., Daughters G.T., Schroeder J.S., Ingels N.B., Alderman E.L.: Exercise response of the denervated heart in long-term cardiac transplant recipients. Am. J. Cardiol. 1980; 46: 213-218
7. Gilbert E.M., Eiswirth C.C., Mealey P.C., Larrabee P., Herrick C.M., Bristow M.R.: β-Adrenergic supersensitivity of the transplanted human heart is presynaptic in origin. Circulation 1989; 79: 344-349
8. Horber F.F., Hoppeler H., Scheidegger J.R., Grunig B.E., Howald H., Frey F.J.: Impact of physical training on the ultrastructure of midthigh muscle in normal subjects and in patients treated with glucocorticoids. J. Clin. Invest. 1987; 79:1181- 1190

18. Future Trends in Pulmonary Rehabilitation

J. MILIC-EMILI

Meakins-Christie Laboratories, McGill University, Montreal, Quebec Canada

During recent years there have been considerable advances in the field of pulmonary rehabilitation.[1, 2] However, the advances have been accompanied by some unfulfilled expectations in areas such as respiratory muscle rest and training. This reflects the fact that pulmonary rehabilitation can probably still be regarded as more of an art than a science. In this connection it should be noted that respiratory muscle fatigue is still in search of a precise definition and of objective criteria to assess its presence and prevalence in stable patients with chronic obstructive pulmonary disease (COPD) or other respiratory disorders.[3] Apart from providing new valuable information, the 1990 meeting "Up-dating on Cardiopulmonary Rehabilitation" has added a new dimension by combining cardiac and pulmonary rehabilitation. Indeed, cardiac and pulmonary abnormalities are often closely linked, as exemplified by dynamic pulmonary hyperinflation. Such linkage was a most refreshing aspect of this meeting.

Although the purpose of the present article, as the title implies, is to point to new directions in pulmonary rehabilitation, I will first briefly assess the present state of this field, with particular emphasis on COPD.

There is irrefutable evidence that home oxygen therapy is safe and prolongs life in hypoxemic COPD patients.[4] However, such treatment does not necessarily improve the quality of life and exercise tolerance.

This is not surprising because in COPD exercise is usually limited by dyspnea associated with levels of ventilation that approach the maximum ventilatory capacity, which is largely determined by the severity of airway obstruction.

By contrast, traditional exercise conditioning improves exercise performance and quality of life, and diminishes dyspnea.[1, 2]

It should be noted, however, that the nature of these responses is still poorly understood.

Fatigue of the respiratory muscles has been suggested as a possible contributor to ventilatory failure and dyspnea in advanced respiratory disease.[5] A corollary of this hypothesis is the possibility that rest may be useful for the treatment of chronic respiratory failure. However, a recent randomized controlled clinical trial of home intermittent negative pressure ventilation in severe but stable COPD patients has failed to demonstrate any clear benefit from resting the respiratory muscles with periodic assisted ventilation.[6] This failure may simply reflect the fact that the population of patients chosen did not exhibit chronic respiratory muscle fatigue, reflecting the fact that respiratory muscle fatigue has yet to be convincingly demonstrated in acute or chronic disease states. Recently developed techniques such as bilateral supramaximal phrenic nerve stimulation show promise for improving the understanding of these conditions.[7, 8] These techniques could also assess the potential benefits of an alternate strategy used for rehabilitation of the respiratory muscles, namely inspiratory muscle training. This approach has also provided controversial results, reflecting non-specific techniques of evaluation, absence of control groups, subthreshold loads, etc.[9]

As indicated above, as yet there are no conclusive results concerning the "best" respiratory rehabilitation program which is to be followed in COPD patients. Probably a specific program should be tailored to each patient depending on his/her status and needs. In this connection, I concur with the views of B. Celli, namely that exercise conditioning should not be limited to the legs with the aim of improving exercise performance, such as increased 12 minute walking distance, but other muscles should also undergo training (e.g. arm exercise).[10] Indeed, in patients with severe COPD it is unsupported arm activities such as brushing teeth that often induce marked dyspnea and tachypnea.[11] Since daily life involves a myriad of arm (and leg) activities, conditioning of the arm muscles appears mandatory to improve the quality of life.

Several modalities of ventilatory support have been recently developed to reduce the work of breathing. Of particular interest is proportional assist ventilation (PAV), a method proposed by Younes et al.[15] The PAV ventilator delivers airway pressure in proportion to patient generated inspired volume, flow or both. In this way, PAV simply reduces the net load against which the inspiratory muscles must work, leaving the muscles, as in normal situations, in full control of breathing pattern (i.e. inspiratory and expiratory durations, tidal volume, flows). This is a clear example of tailoring the pressure support according to the respiratory mechanics and control of breathing of the patient.

Concerning future trends in pulmonary rehabilitation, I think that a distinction should be made between rehabilitation of chronic patients and those in acute ventilatory failure. The latter is probably the area which is most likely to show rapid progress in view of the fact that this condition is presently the object of many investigations. We are now able to better recognize and manage dynamic pulmonary hyperinflation, and by application of continuous positive airway pressure (CPAP) or negative pressure around the thorax it should be possible to manage COPD patients in acute ventilatory failure without the need of intubation[13] and inherent dangers.[12] Although still in its infancy respiratory muscle pharmacotherapy is also of great potential interest.[1,2] A more drastic alternative to rehabilitation is lung transplant which, however, by necessity will only benefit a small number of patients. Rehabilitation of lung transplant patients after surgery is a new area of interest, which will undoubtedly teach us many physiological lessons.

The 1990 meeting in Milan has been an excellent meeting which has stressed the need for more in depth analysis of the present approaches of pulmonary rehabilitation. One important lesson which we have learned is that a given pulmonary rehabilitation approach does not necessarily work in all patients. Clearly, the rehabilitation modality should be tailored according to the needs and framework of each patient. Furthermore, in a given patient the need of improvement may be hierarchical in the sense that the ability to eat and wash may be more important than being able to walk.

Supported by the J.T.C. Memorial Research Fund, the Respiratory Health Networks of Centers of Excellence and the Medical Research Council of Canada

References

1. Make B.J. (Ed.) : *Pulmonary Rehabilitation.* Clinics Chest Med. 1986; 7:(4)
2. Donner C.F. , Bergland E., (Eds.): Advances in pulmonary rehabilitation and management of chronic respiratory failure. Eur. Respir. J. 1989;2:7
3. Macklem P.T.: The importance of defining respiratory muscle fatigue. Am. Rev. Respir. Dis. 1990; 142: 274
4. Anthonisen N.R.: Home oxygen therapy in chronic obstructive pulmonary disease. Clinics Chest Med. 1986; 7: 673-678
5. Macklem P.T., Roussos C.: Respiratory muscle fatigue: a cause of respiratory failure? Clin. Sci. 1977; 53: 419-422
6. Martin J.M., Levy R.D.: Respiratory muscle rest. Problems in Resp. Care 1990; 3: 534-541
7. Bellemare F., Bigland-Ritchie B.: Assessment of human diaphragm strength and activation using phrenic nerve stimulation. Respir. Physiol. 1984; 58: 263-277
8. Aubier M., Murciano D., Lecocguic Y., Viires N., Pariente R.: Bilateral phrenic stimulation: a simple technique in humans. J. Appl. Physiol. 1985; 58: 58-64
9. Grassino A.: Inspiratory muscle training in COPD patients. Eur. Respir. J. 1989; (Suppl. 7): 581-586
10. Sinclair D.J., Ingram O.G.: Controlled trial of supervised exercise training in chronic bronchitis. Br. Med. J. 1980; 1: 519-521
11. Tangi S., Wolf C. R.: The breathing pattern in chronic obstructive lung disease during the performance of some common daily activities. Chest 1973; 97: 126-127

174

12. Grassino A., Rampulla C., Ambrosino N., Fracchia C. (Eds.): *Chronic Pulmonary Hyperinflation.* Verona, Bi & Gi Publishers, London, Springer-Verlag, 1989
13. Milic-Emili J.: Dynamic pulmonary hyperinflation and intrinsic PEEP: consequences and management in patients with chronic obstructive pulmonary disease. Recent Prog. Med. 1990; 81: 733-737
14. Rossi A., Brandolese R., Milic-Emili, J., Gottfried S.: The role of PEEP in patients with chronic obstructive pulmonary disease during assisted ventilation. Eur. Respir. J. 1990; 3: 818-822
15. Younes M., Bilan D., Jury D., Kroker H.: An apparatus for altering the mechanical load of the respiratory system. J. Appl. Physiol. 1987; 62: 2491-2499

Indice analitico

Lightning Source UK Ltd.
Milton Keynes UK
UKOW05f0414081217

314095UK00013B/435/P